UNCOMMON PLANT DRUGS OF AYURVEDA

Indian Medical Science Series No. 35

UNCOMMON PLANT DRUGS OF AYURVEDA

Dr. Gyanendra Pandey

Sri Satguru Publications
A division of
Indian Books Centre
Shakti Nagar, Delhi, INDIA

Sri Satguru Publications
A Division of
Indian Books Centre
40/5, Shakti Nagar,
Delhi-110007 INDIA

First Edition : Delhi, 1994
ISBN 81-7030-404-0

PRINTED IN INDIA

Contents

Acknowledgement : Dr. V.N. Pandey, Director, CCRAS, New Delhi

Assistance : Sumitra Pandey — Ankur Pandey
College of Science, Gurukul Kangri University, Hardwar, U.P.

Prologue

Contribution in the field of medicinal flora, a major part of immense natural resources of country and the wide ranging significance of medicinal plants in the knowledgeable sources of Indian medical science and traditions, by carrying out survey, compilation, collation, study and review of information and data on various aspects of medicinal plants relevant to indigenous medical systems, specially Āyurveda, on potentials of medical and allied importance in plant source of drugs available in India and adjacent regions, with special reference to the facet of plant drugs needy of due attention for utility exhaustively and opening new vistas in multidisciplinary studies and their applied role in resurgence of global interest in the plants used in medicine as herbal cure for the manifold benefit to suffering humanity.

Multiangled and wide purview for taking up the medicinal plants specifically lesser known, newly introduced, unfamiliar or uncommon, recently or imperfectly acquainted, inadequately exploited and getting preminence gradually or diminishing, claimed substitutes-adulterants-varieties-sources of plant drugs and their recurrence, reintroduction and (or) flow towards the current medical practice of Indian medicine having very vast scope, rich sources and extensive spheres of knowledge in reorientation cycle and promotional phases.

Medicobotanical account covering mainly description of plants, taxonomical features, distribution and occurrence, medicinal utility, therapeutic indications, useful parts, relevance in indigenous medicine, allied utility, significance in medicine, Sanskrit names (classical, textual or proposed) and drugs or their kinds concerned and various other aspects and useful informations.

Indices, Lists and Bibliography

Series of material newly focusing plant potentials in applied pattern based on principles and ideology, for covering, adding, supplementing and finally contributing to science and medicine through the studies in Indian medicine, opening with Volume I, containing sections I, II and III, following further presentations.

Families*

1.9	Acanthaceae
2.14,18	Araceae
3.1, 12, 16,17	Asteraceae**
4.6	Caesalpiniaceae
5.7	Cochleospermaceae
6.5, 18	Convolvulaceae
7.8	Cucurbitaceae
8.4, 15	Euphorbiaceae
9.10	Gentianaceae
10.11	Lamiaceae ***
11.18	Rhamnaceae
12.2, 9	Scrophulariaceae
13.6	Verbenaceae
14.3	Vitaceae

---

* Dicotyledonous and Monocotyledonous classes.

** Composiae

*** Labiatae

Code number: Serial number. Sequence of family

Genera

A : 1-10

Acilepis
Adenema
Ageratum
Alectra
Amberoba
Ampelocissus
Ameloveenia
Argyrea
Arisaema
Arum

B : 11-13

Bombax
Bonduc
Bridelia

C : 14-27

Caesalpinia
Canscora
Cardus
Carelia
Cayratia
Centaurea
Clerodendron
Clerodendrum
Cluytia

Species

Adenema hyssopifolium
Ageratum conyzoides
A. houstonianum
A. mexicanum
Alectra parasitica
A. parasitica var. chitrakutensis
A. indicaea
A. avensis
A. cordata
A. orbacchoides
A. sessiliflora
A. thompsoni
Aeschmandra epigenus
Ampelocissus latifolia
A. araneosa
A. arnotiana
A. arneosum
A. tomentosa
A. cordifolium
Atisaema pumilum
Argyrea uniflora
A. bona-nax
A. ornata
Arum guttatum
A. sessiliflorum

Bombax religiosum
Bridelia assamica
B. ovata
B. minutiflora
B. panagiana
B. sacndens
B.montana
B. monatna var. communis
B. retusa
B. retusa var. roxburghiana
B. stipularis
B. crenalata
B. spinosa
B. squamosa

Carelia houstaniana
Cissus araneosus
Cochleospermum religiosum
C. gossyypium
Claxylon mercurialis
Corallocarpus epiegius
Craterostigma plantaginea
Cluytia monoica
Convolvulus candicans
C. hypocrateriformis
Clerodendron spicatum
Clerdendron viscosum
Clerodendrum viscosum
C. infortunatum
C. serratum

C. multiflorum
C. phlomidis
C. castaniaefolium
Caessalpinia digyna
C. oleosperma
Cardus ramosus
C. radicans
Centaurea divaricata
Cicendia hyssopifolia
Cnicus angustifolius

Doronicum calcaratub

Elytraria acaulis
E. acaulis var. acaulis
E. crenata
E. lyrata
Ericoila verticillata
Endestemon viscosus

Glossostylis arvensis
Gentiana verticillata

Hippion orientale
Holmoskioldia sp.
Hymenospermus dentuam

Inula indica
I. vestita

Lamprachaenum micfocophalusm
Lettsomia uniflora

L. ornata

Melasma avense
M. indicum
Micrococa mercurialis
Microlonchus divaricatus

Ocimum aristatum
O. thymiflorum
O. tuberosum
Oligechaeta ramosa
Onopordon lanatum
Orthosiphon glabratus
O. rubicundus
O. pallidus
O. stamineus
O. viscosus
O. grandiflora

Pentanema radiatum
P. vestita
Plectranthes rubicundus

Rivea fragrans
R. hypocrateriformis
R. laotica
R. ornata var. griffthii

Sauromatum venesum
S. guttatum
S. pedatum
Stictophyllum glabrum

Torenia plantaginea
Tragia cannabina
T. hispida
T. involucrata
T. involucrata var. cannabina
T. involucrata var. angustifolia
T. muelleriana var. cordata
T. plukenetii
Tridax procumbens
Tricholepis glaberrima
T. radicans
T. stictophyllum
Tubiflora acaulis
Typhonium scamense
T. orixiens
T. trilobatum

Ventilago calyculata
V. denticulata
V. madraspatana
V. bracteata
V. madraspatana var. calyculata
Vicoa indica
V. auriculata
V. cassini
V. vestita
Volkameria infortunata
Volutarella divaricata
V. remosa

Xeropapus lanugginosus

Indigenous Drugs

Amaravarāyudhāhvaya
Agadakanda
Agnimantha
Araṇī
Arjaka

Bahumūlā
Bandhyāvarī
Bhaṇḍīra
Bhaṇṭāka
Bhṛṅgarāja
Bhṛṅgarāja jāti

Devamañjarī
Dīrghamula

Hastikanda

Kaivarttikā
Karañja
Kaṇṭakīkarañja
Kaṣāyavṛkṣa
Kaṭhiñjara
Kaṭṭīra
Kaṭunāhī
Kaṭunāhītikta
Kuṭheraka

Mārkava

Mūlapatrā

Māmajjaka

Nāhīkanda

Nīlapuṣpī

Nīlimā

Nirguṇḍī

Nirguṇḍībhava vandāka-bandāka

Nirguṇḍī bandāka-vandāka

Lohitā

Lohitayaṣṭikā

Pādaprasarī

Pāṣāṇasaka

Pattaṅga

Phañjī

Pīta bhṛṅgarāja

Raktarodhī

Rakta-vajra-kanda

Sahasramulā

Sukanāsā

Suphalinī

Surendrakanda

Sveta kuṭheraka

Tāmravallī

Vajrakaṇda

Vajraproktā

Vāmataruṇī

Vālanirmūlikā
Vaṭapatra
Vandhyāvarī
Vṛscikālī

Lists partaining to Section I.

Section - I

1

Ageratum conyzoides Linn.

Ageratum cordifolium Roxb

Family: Asteraceae (Compositae)

Regional names: Nilaphuli, Nilam, Gangua (Hindi); Boksuhasal, Gandrbuta, Nathagidu; Dechunty, Uchunti, (Bengala, Osari (Bombay), Pumpilu (Tamil); Tambacoo, Bhakumbhar

Softly hairy annual 1-2 ft. high. Stems branched, terete. Leaves petioled, upto 5 in. long, evate, cuneate to subcordate at the base, crenate. Heads many. small, discoid, arranged in dense terminal corymbs; bracts of involucre linear, acute, ribbed on their backs. Flowers many, the corolla pale blue or white. Achenes angled, often glandular, black; pappus-scales 5, connate below, awned and often barbed.

Flowering and fruiting: January-June, and various months

Distribution: Throughout India, ascending the Himalayas upto 5,000 ft. alt. All the hot countries or tropical regions of world.

Occurring commonly in wastelands, fields, roadsides, banks of canals, streams and irrigated channels, and other various places where abudant often as weed, herbaceous undergrowth and also forming green carpet, and frequently thriving gregariously, in various parts of country from peninsula to hilly regions.

Ageratum conyzoides Linn. Annual, erect, 1-2 ft., or 30-60 cm. tall hispidly hairy; leaves petioled ovate crenate, heads small in dense terminal corymbs, bracts striate acute, ray-fls. many pale blue or white, achenes black, pappus scales 5 awned often serrate below Stems often purplish. Flowers colour varying as heads white, or very pale blue, or very faintly pinkish-purple, also fragrant; corolla white or purple, or pale blue or white.

Ageratum houstonianum Mill.

Carelia houstoniana (Mill.) Kuntze.

Ageratum conyzoides L. var. *mexicana* DC.

Ageratum mexicanum Sims.

Family: Asteraceae

Herb, 16-60 cm. high. Leaves opposite, petiolate, deltoid, lamina 2-10 x 1.5-5.5 cm., crenate-serrate or serrate. Heads discoid, 80-100 flowered, in terminal and axillary dense corymb Involucre biseriate, glandular, greyish hirsute. Corolla violet, infundibuliform, 2.5-3.5 cm. long. Styles branches long, exerting the corolla. Achenes 5-angled, black, hairy, about 2 cm. long, pappus-scales 5, serrate, awn-tipped.

Flowering ad fruiting: November-March

Distribution: Throughout India ascending upto about 1800 m. alt. Most tropical countries in world. Southern India, Central India, Assam, Nilgiri and Pulney hills, Uttar Pradesh, Upper Gangetic Plains, Siwaliks, Bengal; and Nepal.

Ageratum houstonianum Mill. appears to be variety of *Ageratum conyzoides* Linn., and quite similar; and former species may be distinguished by many-flowered, linear heads, linear setaceous, densely hairy involucral bracts and larger corolla than the later species, having distinction mainly of long acurinate involucral bracts in A. *houstonianum* Mill. which islikely to grow in the areas of usual occurrence. of *A. conyzoudes* L. Genus *Ageratum* Linnaeus with about 16 species, probably all American, but now distributed throughout the tropics. Erect herbs or shrubs, glabrous or hairy. erect herbs or under shrubs, aromatic. Leaves opposite or the upper alternate sometimes, petioled, crenate, palmately 3-seriate, oblong-elliptic, acute, herbaceous; receptacle conical, naked or with caducous scales, or flat or nearly so. Corolla tube glandular, sometimes hairy, equal, regular, limb' 5-cleft; Anthers appendaged, base obtuse. Style arms slender, clavate oe elongate. Achenes oblong, 5-angled, glabrous, sometimes hairy along angles; pappus of 5 free or connate scales, or 10-20 narrow unequal scales, lacerate below, long aristate.

Genus *Ageratum* Linn. in family Compositae belonging to tribe Eupatorieae with salient features (heads with the flowers all similar and tubular; anthers subentire at the base; style arms obtuse, papillose; leaves opposite or alternate; corolla rarely orange, never yellow; pappus usually bristly, and subtribe Agerateae with anther-tip appendiculate and achenes 5-angled, and *Ageratum* genera distincts for pappus paleaceous. Tribe Eupatorieae of group 2 Tubuliflorae, with *Ageratum* genus distinguished by heads in dense, terminal corymbs and anthers appendaged at the apex, head with many florets, pappus of 5 scales, herbs aromatic and heads in paniculate corymb.

The leaves, roots, flowers and whole plant of *Ageratum conyzoides* Linn are medicinally useful.

Leaves and flower of the plant contain 0.02% essential oil with powerful nauseating odour; the essential oil containing phenols ester with powerful agreable odour. Oil from African species agreable, consisting almost entirely of a phenolie ester similar in ethyl eugenol.

Leaves of the plant are styptic and applied to cuts and sores, and leaves are externally applied in ague. Juice of roots is antilithic.

Leaves are odoriferous as the leaves when bruised between fingers smell an offensive odour due to presence of some chemical constituents. Essential oil containing phenols (eugenol) 5% and a phenol ester with powerful agreable odour.

The leaves and stem of the plant are useful as fomentation over skin. In eyes affections, the lotion prepared from the leaves after proper decantation is used as eye drop. The infusion of whole plant is useful for diarrhoea internally. It is also used in cases of flatulence and abdominal colie. The juice of the leaves is useful in prolapsus. Leaves and pounded and made into a paste which is applied topically over cuts, bruishes, sores, incised wounds and ulcers as the leaves are styptic for checking the haemorrhage and blood cougulant, and healer and antiseptic for healing the wounds or cuts and other complaints. The juice of leave or a paste of leave when applied over cuts or incised wounds stops the blood and heals the injury.

Leaves are haemostatic, antiseptic and healing in external treatment of wounds, ulcers and sores including injury cuts. Leaves paste is applied to ulcers, burns, boils muscular pains, piles, prolapse of anus, skin affections, ringworm, swelling, snake bite, tumours, hairs lice and scabies. Leaves are useful in uterine disorders, kidney calculus and renal colic, fever, headache, flatulence, colic and other complaints.

Ageratum houstonianum Mill. is also medicinally useful.

Nilpuspī, Raktarodhī and Nīlimā, the Sanskrit names for *Ageratum conyzoides* Linn.

2

Alectra parasitica A. Rich var. chitrakutensis M.A. Rau

The *Alectra parasitica* A. Rich. root parasite plant on the root shrubs or small tree of *Vitex negundo* L., Nirguṇḍī, the host plant, a well-known drug of indigenous systems of medicine.

Family:	Scrophulariaceae
Regional Name:	Gaiya, Midaki

Small root parasite changing black on drying. Stems rhizomatous, perennating with strongly developed underground stem patts, 2.3 cm. thick, horizontally extending with numerous axillary buds in the axills of closely set scale leaves. Rhizome orange-yellow with a stale colour, shrinking considerably on drying. Inflorescense terminal on the rhizome; flower bearing portion of erect axis 5.20 cm. long, angular, purplish, hispid. Leaves very small, mostly scale-like, hispid, largest 0.6 cm. long, linear oblong, obtuse. Racemes rather loose; floral leaves of bracts linear long or longer than the sessile or almost sessile flowers. Bracteoles very slender equally long as calyx tube in open flower, persistent. Calyx campanulate, hairy outside, lobes shorter than the tube, deltoid, acute, Corolla about 1 cm., glabrous, yellow with purple streaks. Filaments short, glabrous, anther cells slightly unequal, obtuse. Ovary globose, style long, inflexed. Capsule globose 0.5 cm. across, splitting into 4-valves. Seeds many, minute, cuneiform.

Flowering & fruting:	September-November; March-June.

Plant found in Uttar Pradesh (Chitrakuta in Banda district) India.

Alectra sessiliflora (Vahl. Kuntz. var. **monticola** (Engl. Melch.

Melasma indicum (Benth.) Wettst. var. *monticolum* Engl.

Alectra indica sensu Hook.f.

Melasma avense (Benth.) Hand.- Mazz.

Annual, rigid herby, hemiparasitic herb, changing black on drying. Leaves opposite or upper ones spirally arranged, sessile or on short petioles, entire, dentate, or deeply incised, ovate-oblong, with cuneate-rounded. cordate base, sparsely pilose, the lower ones 2.4 cm. x 1.2 cm., upper ones small. Flowers yellow, sessile or nearly sessile, in erect, 5.15 cm. long spikes, shorter than bracts, bracteoles ciliate. calyx ovoid, campanulate, angular, pilose,, afterwards inflated, 5-lobed, during anthesis 3.4 mm. long. Corolls yellow, 5.7 mm. long, tube campanulate, lobes, patent, broad subequal the two postetior ones in bud mostly inside. Stamens 4, included, didynamous or subequal anthers 2-celled: anthers cells parallel; stigma thickened or tongue-shaped, entire or shortly 2-lobed Capsule shorter than calyx, subglobose, 4-lobed, enclosed within calyx, loculici dally 2-valved; valves entire or 1-find. Seeds numerous.

Herb found in Dehradun (Sahastradhara) in Uttar Pradesh, India Two species of *Melasma* differ by characterstic distinction, as *Melasma avense* (Benth.) Hand.-Mazz. has ovate-lanceolate, toothed-leaves and sessile flowers, differing from *Melasma thompsani* (Hk.f) Wettst., syn. *Alectra thomosani* Hook.f.

Melasma avense (Benth.) Handel.

Glossostylis avense Benth.

Alectra indica Benth.

Alectra avensis (Benth.) Merrill.

Herb with 6-16 in. stem, naked below, simple or branched above. Leaves sparingly coarsely toothed. Spikes pubescent

3-6 in. Flowers, bracetoles ciliate, calyx 1/2 in. long, yellow lobes, rounded subequal.; filaments ciliate, anthers yellow. Capsule shorter than the calyx, subglobose, 4-lobed. Seeds linear, nucleus very small in the centre of the transparent sausage-shaped testa.

Temperate Himalaya; from Kumaon to Bhutan, altitude 3,000-9,000 ft.; Khasia Mts. altitude 4,000 ft.; Bihar, (top of Parasanath hills).

Distribution: Mauritius

Melasma thompsonii (Hook.f.) Wettst.

Alectra thompsonii Hook. f.

Regional Name: Nirganga

A very singular plant, resembling the South African species *Alectra orbanchoides* Benth. Stems rigid but flexuous, 6-15 in. high, simple or branched of the rootstock, hardly scaberulous, Leaves represented by a few scattened scales 1/10-1/14 in. long, the largest, oblong, obtuse. Racemes 6-10 in., lax fix; bacts minute; pedicels slender. Calyx fruiting hemispheric, 1/4 in. diam; lobes broadly triangular. Capsule globose, as long as the calyx. Seeds as in the A. *indica*, but more minute and elongate- cuneiform.

Bihar, on Parasnath, altitude 3,000 ft.; Maharastra, India.

A parasite also on ***Strobilanthes,, Thomson.***

Alectra indica Benth. Scaberulous, leaves sessile or shortly petioled, ovate-lanceolate or lanceolate, coarsely toothed, base cuneate rarely cordate, bracts longer than the sessile flowers.

A. cordata Benth. (the Himalayan specimens). *Hymenospermus dentuam* Benth. *Glossostylis arvensis* Benth.

Alectra thompsoni Hook.f. Slender, leaves scale-like, flowers racemose, bracts minute.

Genus *Alectra Thunb* species 14, atleast tropical American, African and Indian.-regions; species more in number scattered.

Genus *Alectra* (Tribe: Gerardieae) Calyx-lobes valvate. Anthers 2-celled; leafy herbs, rarely shrub): Calyx campanulate, coupls oblique, spikes braclets.

Genus *Alectra* Thunb. with 30 species in tropical America America, tropical and South Africa and Tropical Asia; the group of small herbs covering 3-4 species in the Himalayas and mountainous regions of Central and Eastern India.

Distinguishing characters of the genus *Alectra* in family (Scrophulariaceae with about 320 genera and 3,000 species) pertains to flower structure as corolla with lower lobes outside in the bud relating to *Alectra* specifically for campanulate calyx of subfoliaceous and 4 stamens in this partial root parasite plants whereas other genera, for the instance with non-parasitic plants and with 2 stamens e.g. *Veronica, Centrathera, Buchnera, Striga* and others).

Alectra sessiliflora (Vahl.) O. Kuntze.

Gerardia sessiliflora Vahl.

Alectra arvensis (Benth.) Merr.

Glossostylis arvense Benth.

Melasma arvense (Benth.) Hand.

Alectra indica Benth.

Erect, scabrid herbs. Leaves sessile or short-petioled, ovate-lanceolate or lanceolate, with acuneate or cordate base, deeply serrate. Flowers in spikes, pale yellow; filaments ciliate; anthers yellow. Capsule shorter than the calyx. Seeds linear, with a transparent, sausage-shaped testa.

Uttar Pradesh, Siwaliks

Alectra parasitica var. *chitrakutensis* Rau occurring in Uttar Pradesh (plant varietal name depicting Chitrakuta, Banda district, U.P.), and various parts of Madhya Pradesh. Parasites herb growing on the roots of generally older shrubs of host plant *Vitext negundo* Linn. *(Verbenaceae)* gregarious in patches flourishing particularly in sandy soils directly exposing to sunlight. and·specially river banks of sandy places suitable for plant growth.

Alectra parasitica var. *chitrakutensis* Rau.

The rhizome of the parasitic plant on the roots of *Vitex negundo* Linn. are mainly medicinally useful, and whole plant and flowering stem are potent.

Rhizomes contain azafrin and flowering stem contains mannitol.

The rhizomes and whole herb are considered useful in treatment of skin diseases, leprosy, leucoderma, skin affections, rheumatism and debility. Rhizome of the plant are specifically useful as an effective drug in leucoderma.

The decoction and powder of rhizome of herb are internally useful in treatment of leucoderma mainly and also useful in allied skin diaseases and leprotic ailments, and in other dermatological complaints. It is given in rheumatism and also as tonic.

The small root parasite on shrub of *Vitex negund* Linn. found in particular areas with confined or varying occurrence in some parts of country (such as Madhya Pradesh, Uttar Pradesh, Maharastra, Bihar and others) may be collected during the March-April and in the time of availability in different areas of restricted growth.

Nirgundi, the host plant *Vitex negundo* Linn. is major drug of Indigenous medicine.

Nirguṇḍī Vandāka, or Bandāka the Sanskrit name for the plant *Alectra parasitica* A. Rich var. *chitrakutensis* M.A. Rau

Nirguṇḍi bhava bandākaṁ: Kākacaṇḍīsvạra Karpatandram, Vandāka kalpa.

3

Ampelocissus latifolia (Roxb.) Planch

Vitis latifolia Roxb.

Vitis montana Lawson.

Ampolocissus latifolia Planch.

Family: Vitaceae

Regional names: Panibel, Dokarbel, Amlosa, Musal (Hindi), Govila (Bengla), Golinda (Marathi), Karantavalli (Malayalam), Kattukkodimundirigai (Tamil), Bedasativva (Telgu), Bechhuti, Belparsua, Dhamado, Hasualarange, Pitehidita.

Large climber, very glabrous except the young parts of climber. Stems hollow, striate. Leaves long-petioled, 3-7 ft. long, orbicular-cordate, 3-7-angled or lobed, lobes dentate; basal nerves 5. Peduncles long, bifureate, one of the branches consisting usually of a slender forked tendril. Flowers small, reddish-brown, in small compact thyrsoid cymes; pedicels often equalling the flowers; petals 5, distinct, style very short or O. Berry about the size of a currant, black, 2-seeded. Seeds elliptic, margins transversely rugose.

Sub-Himalayan tract from Sutelaj eastwards to Kumaon upto, also in Chota Nagpur, Central and Southern India; Assam Sylhet, Konkan, Western Ghats from Bombay to the Nilgiris and Anamalais, Deecan, Carnatic, North Cirears and other regions Siwalik ranges and the and the sal forests, and Rohilkhand, Oudh, Merwara, Madhya Bharat, Bundelkhand, Brijbhumi in Uttar Pradesh and other areas in India.

Ampelocissus latifolia (Roxb.) Planch. Whole plant quite glabrous; leaves roundly cordate, 3-7 angled or lobed, peduncle shortisk, bearing slender forked tendril, petals distinct; flowers small, reddish-brown.

Stems weak, hollow, far-climbing, striate, generally quite glabrous; leaves 6-8 by 6-8 in., glossy; flowers very small, in small somewhat compact thyrsoid cymes; fruit the size of a currant black, 2-seeded; seeds small, elliptical, with a linear tubercle on the back and the margins transversely rugose, bluntly ridged on the face. Species distinctively with flowers paniculately cymose- *Vitis latifolia* Roxb. North-West India, Konkan and Coromandal coast southwards.

Ampelocissus tementosa (Roth.) Planchon.

Vitis tomentosa Heyne ex Roth.

Vitis lanata wall.

Vitis ternata, Reyna.

Vitis cinnamomea Wall.

Regional Names: Ghoralidi (Santhal),

Atukulabaddu (Telgu),

Sirunaralai (Tamil),

Baliakand, Deblia,

Kumharlat

Whole plant covered with a thick wooly persistent tomentum, leaves palmate 3-5-angled or lobed, flowers sessile in shortly peduncled compact densely wooly cymes.

Plant usually covered with cinnamoneus wool. Leaves upto 7-15 x 5-18 cm., orbicular, cordate, often 3-5-lobed, serrate, drying brown below. Flowers red, or ssarlet, turning dark brown when drying, showing conspicously in the midst of the white woolly tomentum. Peduncles 3-6 in. Stout, woody, bearing a stiff wooly, forked tendril 1 in. below the cymes. Fruit berry, 1/3 in., black, round. Seeds 1/3 by 1/4 in. broadly oblong, flat, the margin ineurved, the face with a thick rounded ridge running down the middle, pale.

Western Peninsula, from Canara southwards. South-West India, common in open serub and deciduous forests in the plains and upper Ghats, Karnataka in India.

Ampelocissus araneosus (Dalz. & Gibs.) Planch.

Ampelocissus aurneosa *Planch*
Gissus araneosus Dalz. & Gibs.
Vitis araneosus (Dalz. Gibs.) Lawson.
Regional Names: Kamraj (Hindi)
Bendervel (Bombay)
Chamarmusti,

Whole plant covered with a deciduous down, except on the upper surface of the leaves where it is persistent. Stems flattened or slender, far-climbing. Leaves 4-6 in., membraneous terminal leaflets elliptic, lateral semi-elliptic; petiole 1-2 in. ; leaflets shortly, stalked, serrate, at length.

Western Peninsular part of India; hoghest Ghats of Konkan (Concan); Southern India.

Ampelocissus araneesa (Dalz. & Gibs.) Planeh. resembles with *Ampelocissus divaricata* (Wall ex Lawson) Planch. syn. *Vitis divaricata* Wala. ex Lawson. in regard to flowers and fruits; and both species with petals and stamens 5; as allied to V. tementosa but sufficiently differs in the composition and texture of leaves in the plant.

Ampelocissus arnotiana Planch.

Vitis indica sensu Lawson.
Ampelocissus arnotiana Planch.
Vitis erioelada W. & A.
Vitis rugosa Wall.
Vitis indica W. & A.

Regional names:
Amoluka (Bengla),
Jangli-angur (Hindi),
Randraksha (Marathi),
Semparavalli (Malayalam),
Sambarvalli (Tamil-Telgu),

Plant with stout stem, cylindrical, slender, permanently woolly. Branches, leaves and peduncles covered with a dense woolly tomentum. Leaves glabrous at length and shining above, cordate-ovate, acute, denticulate-serrate, points of the curvatures hard almost spiny. Peduncles stoutish, bearing a long simple. Flowers in short cylindric spikes about 2 in. Fruit globos, the size of a large currant, 2-4 seeded. Seeds 1/8-1/4 in., eliptic, slightly curved on the back from end to end, otherwise flatish, with a spathulate tubercle, the wedge-shaped; berry purple.

Species very closely allied to *Vitis erioclada* W. & A. in general appearence, and *Vitis indica* Mig. shows distinction.

Western Peninsula, from the Konkan southwards. Central India, Uttar Pradesh, Madhya Pradesh; Southern India, extending to Ceylon.

Genus *Vitis* Linn.-about 230 or 375 species growing mostly in the tropics and subtropics of Asia, Africa and Polynesia, more rarely in America; around 75 or more in India (including cultivated species also) specially in the north-west); and about 11 or more in the upper gangetic plains in Central India and allied regions. (*Vitis* Linn. large genus of the of sarmantose shrubs, climbing usually by leaf-opposed tendrils, rarely booting, species coming (generic, species and cultivars etc.) under *Ampelocissus* Planch, *Vitis* Linn., *Cissus* Linn., *Cayratia* A. Juss. and other genera in Vitaceae (Ampelideae).

The roots, fruits, root bark and whole plant of *Ampelocissus latifolia* (Vahl.) Planch. sysn. *Vitis latifolia* Roxb. are medicinally useful.

Roots of the plant *Ampelocissus latifolia* Planch. are useful in the wounds and ulcers.

Roots of the plants *Ampeloeissus latifolia* Planch. are topically applied over the wounds.

Roots of the plant *Ampelocissus araneosa* Planch. are cooling and astringent.

The juice of roots of the olant *Ampelocissus arnottiana* Planch. are useful, with kernel of coconut, employed as a depurative and aperient. The juise is used as alterative in form of decoction; and useful as blood purifier and diuretic particularly helping in healthy urination.

The roots of *Ampelocissus latifolia* Planch. are pounded and externally applied over wounds and fresh injuries. Roots are ground and made a paste which is applied to fractures, sprains, bruises, injuries, wounds and ulcers. For the application of paste on bone fractures, the bandage on the effected part properly provided suitable in bone fracure cases.

The roots are useful in dysentery, fever, menstrual disorders and stomach troubles. Whole plant is useful in snake-bite and pnuemonia. Roots are useful as galactogogue. Roots are externally applied to inflammation or swellings. Fruits are edible.

The roots of the plant *Ampelocissus arnotiana* Planch syn. Vitis indica Lawson. are made into a paste and applied externally to swellings, wounds and sores.

The roots or tubers, stesm and fruits are medicinally useful of the plant *Ampelocissus barbata* (Wall.) Planch. sys. *Vitis barbata* Vahl. The roots are externally useful in eczema, swellings and wounds. Fruits are edible.

The roots and whole plant of *Ampelocissus tomentosa* Planch syn. *Vitis tomentosa* Heyne. are medicinally useful. The roots are useful in boils, sprains, skin affections, eczema, wounds, sores, veneral diseases, anasarca, carbuncle, bones fractures, dropsy, dysentery, neural pains in lower limbs, pleurisy, pneumonia, puerpureal fever, sores, spleenic disorders, swellings, tubercles, fistula and other complaints. In these complaints, the roots and whole plant are used in different forms and relevant usage which include internal and external applications.

Hastikanda, the Sanskrit name for *Ampelocissur latifolia* Planch.

4

Bridelia crenulata Roxb.

Bridelia roxburghiana (Mueller) Gehrm.

Bridelia retusa Sprengel. var. *roxburghiana* Mueller.

Family: Euphorbiaceae

Small deciduous trees: shoots brown-teemntose. Blade 4-12 x 2-5 cm., elliptic-oblong, obtuse, subcordate below: main nerves 22-24 pairs, with parallel cross nerves connecting them. Disc reddish. Drupe globose, turning black.

Flowering and fruiting: March-August

Common in plains and upper Ghats, mainly in deciduous forests in Peninsular India.

Bridelia scandens (Roxb.) Willd.

Cluytia scandens Roxb.

Family: Euphorbiaceae

Scandent shrubs. Leaves 5-14x 2.5-7 cm., elliptic, rounded, subcordate below, glabrous; main nerves about 14-pairs, with parallel cross nerves of leaves. Disc without bristles. Drupe globose, turning black.

Flowering and fruiting: November-March

Commonly growing in Ghats in outer areas of semi-evergreen forests if Western Peninisula in India.

Both species of *Bridelia* Willd. may be distinguishable on the basis of habit and flowers mainly as *Bridelia crenulata* Roxb. is erect tree with flowers axillary and clustered, whereas *Bridelia scandens* (Roxb.) Willd. is scandent shrub with flowers in interrupted and false spikes.

Bridelia retusa Spreng.

Bridelia spinosa Willd.

Family: Euphorbiaceae

Regional Names: Khaja, Kaj, Kaja, Lamkana, Gaya, Ekdania Gondni (Hindi), Mukhayini (Malayalam), Asana (Marathi), Geio, Kantakoi (Bengla), Phatarphod (Bombay), Benth-yepi (Telugu), Mullavenagi (Tamil).

Small or moderate-sized erect deciduous tree, more or less spinescent when young; bark geey. Leaves coriaceous, elliptic-oblong, ovate or obovate, acute, obtuse or rounded at the apex, the base usually rounded, bright-green, and glabrous on the upper surface and turning pinkish-purple before falling, often finely tomentose beneath; main lateral neyves 15-25 pairs, straight, prominent, finely reticulate between; petioles 1/4-1/2 in. long, stipules ovate-lanceolate, unequal at the base, deciduous. Flowers dioecious, greenish-yellow,sessile or shortly pedicelled, arranged in dense axillary clusters or in long axillary or terminal panicled spikes exceeding the leaves; bracts small, obtuse, villous. Calyx 1/8 in. in diam., lobes fleshy, spreading, triangular-ovate, acute, glabrous and often tinged with red, tube pubescent. Petals of males obovate,_ pectinate; females subspathulate. Disc male fl. thick and pulpy; females truncate, enclosing the ovary. Drupes fleshy, subglobose, 1/3 in. diam., seated on the persistent hardly enlarged calyx, flesh-coloured or purplish-black when mature or quite ripe.

Flowering and fruiting: May-July and cold season (fruits ripen).

Distribution: Outer Himalayan ranges from Kashmir to Mishmi upto 3,500 ft. alt.) and southwards to Southern India and Ceylon, extending to Burma and Malacca.

Occurring abundantly in the Upper Gangetic plains; Siwalik range, Bundelkhand, Rohilkhand Sub-Himalayan tracts, Madhya Pradesh, Uttar Pradesh, North Oudh, Rajputana, and other areas. Throughout India frequently in varying extents.

Bridelia montana Willd.

Bridelia montana var. *communis* Prain.

Bridelia montana Royale. (not of Willd.)

Family: Euphorbiaceae

Regional names: Gondani, Kargnalia, Gondi (Hindi),

Asano (Bombay), Pantegi (Telgu),

Vengaimaram (Tamil), Kaisho (Assam),

Small or moderate-sized glabrous deciduous tree; trunk short, with a low spreading crown; bark grey dark; branchlets often warted. Leaves membranous, very variable, 4-7 in. long, obovate-oblong, or broadly obovate, obtuse acute or abruptly mucronate, entire, often shining above, paler beneath, but not glaucous; main laternal nerves 8-15 pairs, slightly arched; petioies 1/10-1/4 in. long, stipules deciduous. flowers monoecious, small, greenish-yellow, shortly pedicelled and arranged in dense axillary clusters; bracts many, very short, ciliate; calyx 1/8-1/4 in. indiam; lobes triangular-ovate, not enlarging in fruit; potals broadly ovate, entire. Fruit 1/3 in long of nearly, ovoid-oblong or fusiform.

Flowering and fruiting : April-May or summers

Distribution : Sub-Himalayantracts from the Jhelum eastwards, Khasia Hills, Madhya Pradesh, Bihar and Orissa. Upper Burma.

Upper Gangetic plains, Siwalik range, North Oudh forests and other adjoining areas.

Bridelia stipularis Blume Syn. *Bridelia scandens* Willd. Large more or less scandent evergreen shrub with dark-grey or brownish bark. Stem 2-8 in. in diam.; branches often with long deflexed spines, the young shoots pubescent or fulvous-tomentose. Leaves subcoriaceous, 2-6 in. long, elliptic-oblong or obovate, obtuse or subacute, round or cordate at the base, glabrous or pubenlous above, fulvous-tomentose beneath, margins sometimes undulate or repand; main lateral nerves 8-12 pairs, slightly arching, the transverse veins parallel and right angles, petioles 3/8 in. long. Flowers monoecious, greenish-yellow, in small dense axillary cluster or long spikes, often subtender by hairy obliquely ovate-lanceolate acute stipule like bracts1/8 in. long; male flowers sessile, female fls. pedicelled, pubescent or glabrate; calyx 1/8 in. diam., distinctly enlarging in fruit, lobes connate below, lanceolate-acuminate; petals 1/10 in. long., suborbicular, shortly cuneate at the base, crenulate towards the apex. Drupe nearly 1/2 in. long, oblong, obtuse, smooth, bluish black and juice when ripens.

Distribution: Threughout the hotter parts of India and in Ceylon, extending to Burma and to the Malay Peninsula and Islands. Sub-Himalayan tracts, sal forests of Oudh, Upper Gangetic plains adjoining areas.

Distinguishing characters of the species mainly of habit, leaves, flowers and fruits: *Bridelia retusa* Spreng. Small tree with stout more or less persistent spines; flowers dioecious; leaves deciduous, main lateral nerves 15-20 pairs straight, prominent; drupe globose; when flowers monoecious leaves persistent and nerves more or less arching in small tree of *Bridelia montana* var. *communis* Prain.

Genus *Bridelia* Willdenow with species about 30, in tropical Asia, Africa and Australia, falls in family Euphorbiaceae (species about 4,000 throught the world chiefly tropical). Genus *Bridelia* Willd. with salient features of woody shrubs or trees; leaves often with parallel main veins, alternate, quite entire, sometimes with strong straight nerves and prominent veins; flowers (usually) dioecious or monoscious, small or minute, arranged in axillary or spicate culsters, sessile or very shortly pedicelled, bracts small, scale-like; male flowers numerous and female flowers few or solitary (with other characters); disc double, the inner forming a membranous central truncate cone often enclosing the young ovary, cupular in male and usually with an inner corona enclosing ovary in female; ovary 2-locular (rarely 3-celled), glabrous; ovules 2 per locules; styles 2, free or shortly united below, forked or subentire; stigmas deeply 2-fid; fruits small drupes, usually globose, with one or two usually 1-seeded cocci or pyrenes; seeds with usually fleshy sometimes membranous albumen and thin or fleshy cotyledons. Genus *Bidelia* Willd. distinguishing from other relevant geners on the basis of specific characteristics of habit, leaves, flowers and fruits in comparison.

Two main species *Bridelia retusa* Spmeng. and *Briddlia verrucosa* Haines are recognisable by salient features. *Briddelia retusa* Spreng. is a large tree; leaves rigidly coriaceous, with straight nerves; bracteoles few, coriaceous; calyx enlarged in fruit. Throughout the Siwaliks and sub-Himalayan tract in Uttar Pradesh, specially in the moister parts ad often associate with sal forests in October to January. Sapwood yellowish-white, heartwood grey or olive-brown, hare, compact, even-and close-grained, seasons well, annual rings distinct. Wood is quite useful in economic or commercial purposes. Bark is used for tanning. The ripe fruit is sweetish and eaten, and the leaves are used for cattle-feed as fodder.

Bridelia verrocosa Maines. is a small tree; leaves membranous, with more or less arcuate nerves; bracteoles numerous, membranous; calyx not enlarged in fruit. It is fairly common in ravines or banks of rivers (upto 3,500 ft. alt.) specially in the Siwaliks and sub-Himalayan tracts in Uttar Pradesh. Woods mottled, otherwise very similar to former species, also used economically to some extents in smaller size. Leaves are lopped for cattle fodder, fruits are not eaten. It flowers and fruits during November-April.

Various important species of the genus *Bridelia* Willdenow:

Bridelia squamosa (Lamk.) Gaertn.

Bridelia retusa sensu Hook. f.

Cluytia squamosa Lamk.

Bridelia monoica (Lour.) Merrill.

Chuytia monoica Lour.

Bridelia tomentosa Bl.

Bridelia crenulata Roxb.

Bridelia retusa var. *rexburhiana* Muell.-Arg.

Bridelia roxburghiana (Muell.-Arg.) Gehrm.

Bridelia ovata var. crustisii (Hook.f.) Airy Shaw.

Bridelia crustisii Hook. f.

Bridelia penangiana Hook. f.

Bridelia minutiflora Hook. f.

Bridelia assamica Hook. f.

Bridelia verrucosa Haines.

Bridelia montana auct. non Willd.

Bridelia seandens (Roxb.) Willd.

Cluytia scandens Roxb.

Bridelia stipularis sensu Hook. f.

Bridelia squamosa (Lamk.) Gehrmann.

Cluytia squamosa Lamk.

Bridelia retusa sensu Hook. f.

The species of *Bridelia* genus have medicinal, economic, and commercial and kinds of utility to varying extents and in regard to certain species in particular. The roots, bark, fruits and leaves of the plants are medicinally useful and employed in various therapeutic and allied purposes, on account of their medicinal efficacy.

The plant *Bridelia montana* Willd. is anthelmintic. The roots and bark are astringent. They contain tannin. The bark of the plant *Bridelia retusa* Spreng. contains tannin 16-40%; the roots and bark are astringent; and bark with gingili oil used as liniment in rheumatism.

The fruits of various plants of *Bridelia squamosa Bridelia assamica* (Gaertn. (Lank.), Hook. f., *Bridelia scandens* (Roxb.) Willd. and *Bridelia retusa* Spreng. are edible.

The stem bark of *Bridelia crenulata* Roxb. is considered useful in birth control and similarly the bark of *Bridelia squamosa* (Lamk.) Gaertn. is useful as antifertility plant.

The bark of *Bridelia squamosa* (Lamk.) Gaertn. is useful as an astrigent drug in various ailments. The bark is applied over cuts, wounds and tubercle affections. The bark is useful in diarrhoea, general debility, earache, waist pain or backache, snake bite and other complaints. The bark is also useful in rheumatism. The leaves and fruits are useful in stomach troubles specially in stomachache. The fruits are laxative, and useful in constipation.

The plant *Bridelia squamosa* (Lamk.) Gaertn. is also useful in veterinary medicine, and leaves as fodder for cattles.

Suphalinī, Kaṣāyavṛkṣa, the sanskrit names for the plant drug.

5

Caesalpinia digyna Rottl.

Caesalpinia oleopserms Roxb.

Family: Caesalpiniaceae (Leguminoseae sub-family)

Regional names: Bakerimula, Vakeri-mul (Hindi), Umul-kuchi (Bengla), Vekri-mula (Bombay), Nune-gacca (Telugu), Vakribhayu (Gujarati), Vakeri, Vakeri ca bhata (Marathi), Nuni-gatcha (Tamil).

Large much branched prickly straggling shrub. Leaves up to 30 cm. long, leaflets close, oblong, obtuse, sessile. Flowers bright pale yellow, 1-5-1.8 cm. across, in supra.axillary racemes with length about 7-20 cm. Paas 2-4.6 cm. long, oblong, thick, fleshy, crowned by the long persistent style. Flowering and fruiting: Cold season or October-February

Distribution: Eastern Himalaya, Eastern and Western Peninsula, Burma,- Ceylon, Malaya. Gujarat, Maharastra, Konkan, Assam,- and Bengal in India.

Cenus *Caesalpinia* Linnaeus in family Caesalpiniaceae R.B. (about 152 genera with over 2,800 species in tropics and sub-tropics, abundant in America; anc about 23 genera and 80 species in India) with salient features-Armed climbing shrubs or trees. Leaves bipinnate. Outer sepals slightly larger. Petals usually yellow. Stamens declinately; filaments villous mm at base. Ovary sessile, few-ovuled; style usually persistent Pods oblong or obvoid, not winged, subturgid, beaked by style.

Salient features of the genus *Caesalpinia* Linn. (species about 40 widely spread in the tropics of both hemispheres) in general—Robust erect trees, shrubs or woody prickly climbers. Leaves large, abrnutly bipinnate. Flowers showy, yellow, in copious axillary racemes. Calyx deeply cleft, with the disk confined to its base, the lobes imbricated, the lowest the largest, cucullate. Petals spreading, usually orbicular with a distinct claw, the uppermost smaller that the others. Stamens 10, free, declinate; anthers oblong; uniform, versatile. Ovary sessile or subsessile, few-ovuled; style filiform, sometimes clubbed at the tipe; stigma terminal. Pod oblong or ligukate, thin and flat, or thicker and subturgid, indehiscent or dehiscent, smooth or all over with wiry spines.

Various important species of the genus *Caesalpinia* Linn.:

Caesalpinia crista L.

Caesalpinia ponduc (L.) Roxb.

Guilandina bonduc L.

Caesalpinia bonducella (L.) Fleming.

Caessalpinia crista Linn.

Caesalpinia bonduc Roxb.

Caesalpinia major (Medik.) Dandy & Excell.

Bonduc majos Medik

Caesalpinia bonduc sensu Roxb. *non Guilandia bonduc* L.

Caesalpinia nuga (Linn.) Ait.

Caesalpinia sepiaria Roxb.

Caesalpinia coriaria (Jacq.) Willd.

Caesalpinia cacullata Roxb.

Mezonevron cuclkatum (Roxb.) W. & A.

Caesalpinia decapetala (Roth. Alston.

Reichardia decaoetala Roth.

Caesalpinia sepiria Roxb.

Caesalpinia spicata Dalz.

Wagatea spicata (Dalz.) W.

Moullava spicata (Dalz.) Nicolson.

Almeloveenia spinosa Dennst.

Caesalpinia mimosoides Lamk.

The roots of plant *C. digyna* contain vakerin, a crystalline compound in 3% yield. Pod-cases containing taniin but not in seeds; bitter substance bonducin, saponin found.

A crystaline phenolic substance, provisionally named as vikerin insolted from the root of plant; earlier with its molecular formula C_{15} H_{18} O_{10} and later modified correctly as C_{14} H_{16} O_8.; Vakerin m.p. 238^6. On acetylation with acetic anhydride in pyridine or in the presence of fused Na-acetate, vakerin gave a penta-acetyl derivative having m.p. 205^0 With diazomethane, dimethyl ether, m.p. 199^6. The dimethyl other on acetylation with acetic anhydride in presence of a drop of perchloric acid gave triacetyl vakerin dimethyl ether, with m.p. 130°. After revision of molecular formula of vakerin, it contained one methoxyl and five hydroxyl groups which include two phenolic. Physical and chemical characteristics of vakerin found to be identical with those of bergenin and the identity further confirmed by IR spectra in phytochemical screening of vakerin, the principle isolated mainly from plant *Caesalpinia digyna* Rottl. which is popularly known as Vakeri-mula or similar names, and the active crystalline phenolic substance vakerin found in its roots, named similarly.

Roots of *Caesalpinia cista* Linn. and its powder not showing any flourescence when exposed to ultraviolet, but the extract in one per cent NaOH solution, ethyl alcohol and solvent ether emitted a light green fluorescence under ultraviolet light. The seeds of plant are globular, shiny and grey with thick testa and ex-albuminous. Transection of seeds showing a palisade layer composed or vertical, columnar and laterally close appressed cells. Thickenings present on the walls of palisade cells, appearing as 6-12 denticulate projections, in tangential section, into the lumen cells. Palisade layer followed by a layer of brearer cells and thick zone of parenchyamtous cells. Majority of the bearer cells I-T shaped in this species, non-lignified and thick-walled. Structure of epidermal as well as mesophyll cells of the cotyledons with their contents also form very conspicous features. Powder of the seeds slide microscopically shows columnar palisade cells, bone-shaped thick walled cells, small roundish to polygonal bearer cells, starch grains and other. Those characters in macerations and powder form proving helping aids in pharmacognostically identifying the species of *Caesalpinia* and other plant specimens. Biological investigations on pharmacological activity of plant show various efficiency in different parts of species from *Caesalpinia* used medicinally.

Powdered seeds of *Caesalpinia crista* Linn. found with anti-estrogenic activity in mice and rabbits; and the anti-fertility action of seeds noted in mice and rats. Nuts of the plant found to have significant anti-diarrhoeal activity in mice; and the effect of drug coult not be attributed to tannins as nuts devoided of tannin. Alcoholic extracts of the roots and stem of this species shows anti-viral activity against Vaccinia virus; and the extract of roots of *Caesalpinia sepiaria* Roxb. found with anti-viral activity against both Ranikhet disease virus and vaccinia virus, during screening of plants for biological activity.

A bitter substance, bonducin, isolated from the plant; seeds contain bitter substance phytosterinin, bonducin, saponin, fatty oil 20-24%, starch, sucrose, two phytosterols; the oil contains ineffective against bird malaria.

Caesalpinia nuga (Linn.) Ait. yields a fish poison in its pulped fruit and stems. Other species C. *sappan* Linn.

contain essential oil in leaves 0.16-0.25%, brasilin, d-x-phellandrene as the chief constituent; and oscimene also found; Pod-cases and bark with tannin.

Caesalpinia genus has some important species with medicinal efficacy. *Caesalpinia nuga* (Linn.) Ait. roots diuretic, tonic, and useful in gravel and stone in urinary bladder. Leaves of *Caesalpinia sepiaria* Roxb. emmenagogue, laxative and applied to burns; and its roots purgative. Powder of pods from *Caesalpinia coriaria* (Jacq.) Willd. astringent, tonic and antiperiodic. Decoction of pods useful in treating the bleeding piles; and decoction of bark antiperiodic and useful in chronic fever.

Caesalpinia spicata Dalz. (Karingi) fruits useful as powder or decoction in bodyache, general debility and as tonic recipe. Memangiakskel, the plant known as *Caesalpinia cuculata* Roxb., considered useful against cramps, convulscence and other parts medicinally useful of this plant. *Caesalpinia decapelata* (Roth.) Alston., the plant (Karangs, Kather) as decoction or powder useful in jaundice; and also for veterinary use of decoction employed as mouth-wash in animals suffering from mouth saves. The paste or decoction of stem, of *Caesalpinia mimesoides* Lamk. (Timulu, Kilansadu) useful for external application.

Caesalpinia pulcherrima Linn., now known as *Poinciang pulcherrima* Linn. (Guletura, Puraiphul, Sandhesaro, Mayuram, Krishachura, Ratnagandhi) useful medicinally as its leaves stimulant, emmenagogue and purgative; bark emmenagogue and abortifacient; flowers useful against bodyache in form of infusion or expressed juice; and the infusion of flowers pectoral and febrifuge, and useful in bronchitis, asthma and malarial fevers. Seeds useful in gum complaints and ringworm and fresh leaves of this plant, generally grown in gardens throughout country, contain HCN, and leaves also useful in ailments, and as stimulant.

Caesalpinia digyna Rottl. popularly known as Vakeri-mul, is efficacious medicine for various ailments particularly for pthisis, scrofulous affect'ons and diabetes. Roots are astringents and containing active substance vakerin. Roots and leaves are both mainly useful medicinally. Leaves expressed juice and roots powder in average doses of 5 ml. and 3-6 gms. respectively indicated; and rects are applied as paste or after grinding (rubbing) externally and also internally given in mixing into water of about a cup or few teaspoon ful. This is therapeutic use in uleers, scrofulous ailments, abscess, fistula, glandular complaints with pus formation and similar ailing conditions of ulcerations, lymphatic adenoids, chronic wounds or ulcers and inflammation of lymphatic glands. The roots or knots are frequently given as useful remedy in the treatment of chronic ulcers of various kinds and also suggested in bone tuberculosis and tubercle glands for long usage. The roots of plant are Vranasodhana, Vraṇaropaṇa, Balya and Kaṇḍūghna, Kaṭupauṣṭika and Tikta; and useful in treatment of Vraṇa, Nāḍīvraṇa, Bhagandara, Duṣṭavraṇa, Gaṇḍamālā, Kuṣṭha, Premeha, Krimi, Arsa and other diseases. Mainly the plant drug with certain properties-Tikta rasa, Uṣṇa vīrya, Kaṭu-vipāka, laghu guṇa, Vātakapha Sāmaka and other properties and actions in various therapeutic uses.

Aṅgāravallī and Karañjī, the kind of Karanja (Madanapāla Nighaṇṭu and Kaiyadeva Nighantu, auṣadhi varga, 969-970).

Other two kinds of Karanja-Kaṇṭakarrahja and (Kuberākṣa) and Pūtikarṅja (Ghṛtakaranja), the major indigenous drugs with source plants.

Caesalpinia crista Linn. and *Pengamia pinnata* (Linn.) Merr. Plant *Caesalpinia sappan* Linn. source for another indigenous drug Pattaṅga (Bakam).

6

Clerodendrum viscosum Vent.

Clerodendron infortunatum auct. non. L.

Clerodendron infortunatum L.

Volkameria infortunata Roxb.

Volkoameria infortunata Roxb.

Clerodendron viscosum Vent.

Clerodendron cordatum Den.

Clerodendron castaneaefolium Klotzsch.

Family: Verbenaceae

Regional names: Bhant, Kaur, Kadu (Hindi), Bakada (Telgu), Angara (Tamil), Bhat (Bombay), Perugilai (Tamil), Gurrapukattiyaku (Telgu), Peruku (Malayalam), Bhat (Bengla), Kari (Marathi), Kalibasut (Punjab), Pumiaye, Addakajo, Ghato, Nayibera.

Shrub upto 12 ft. high or around 4 ft. usually, often gregarious, softly tomentese shrub or small tree sometimes, yellow white-villous upwards; branchlets bluntly 4-angular or branches acutely quadrangular towards apex. Leaves entire, ovate, shortly acuminate, cordate, 4-10 in. or 16x12 cm. long, entire or denticulate (lvs. sometimes varying in South and North), and elsewhere, sparingly hairy on both sides, base cordate or rounded, thickly chartaceous, cordate or obtuse, lvs. from round-ovate to broad-oblong, somewhat roughly hairy above, beneath densely villous or thinly hairy often with small obscure round glands; ventation subpalmate; petiole 1-4 in. long, hairy, cylindric. Flowers on rather long, terminal panicle; panicles 6-12 by 4-8 in., erect, branchiate, sometimes leafy on the main rachis, upper branches and calyces more or less reddening, panicle length upto 20 cm., with densely pubescence; bracts conspicuous, leaf-like deciduous bracts of the cymes usually caducous; flo. usually white tinged with pink or varying colour. Corolla densely hairy outside, white, upto 2 cm. long, white tinged with pink or bluish purple, pubescent; tube 1 cm. long, slender; lobes longer than tube. subequal, spreading, obtuse. Calyx 1/2 in. long (in fls.), segments divided to the base, 5-partite, silky-pubescent, much enlarged in furit, segments broadly lanceolate, very acute, suberect. Filaments glabrous. Drupe 1/3 in. or around, seated on the enlarged pink calyx, 1/3 in diam., sub-globose, purple black when ripens.

Flowering and fruiting: April-May; December-April; and various or almost seasons.

Distribution: Throughout India from Himalayas (4,000 ft. alt.) and Assam to Ceylon, Singapore, Burma, Malaya and in the warm regions; Indomalaysia.

Plant occurring commonly throughout India, the Sub-Himalayan tracts from the Jamuna eastwards, also in, Marwara (Rajasthan), Bundelkhand, Madhya Bharat, Bengal, North-West India, Southern and Central India, outer Himalayan ranges, U.P. hills Upper Gangetic plains, Siwaliks, Punjab, Karnatka, Peñiñsular ghats and other provinces and areas; often as an under growth in forests and in open places, and near populated or rural vicinties. Plant also cultivated as a hedge shrub.

Genus *Clerodendrum* Linn. in the family Verbenaceae (species about 700, chiefly in the tropical regions of both hemispheres), belonging to tribe 3 Viticeae (Inflorescence cymose, centrifugal, cymes panicled, drupe with usually pyrens, and tree or shrubs), has specifically main characters such as corolla 2-lipped, stamens didynamous, leaves simple or digitate and further signify the characterstic of drupe with four 1-seeded pyrens; and distinguishing characters of flowers calyx campanulate, limb truncate, or 5-toothed or almost 5-partite, separates this genus from *Holmskioldia* Retz. with calyx in flower large, patelliform, calyx rotate, widely patent, entire or obscurely 5-lobed; Similarly the genus *Premna* Linn. distinguishable by stamens not much exserted and pyrene one 4-seeded, as both genera (*Clerodendrum* and *Premna)* have calyx without any glands and corolla limb slightly oblique.

Clerodendrum viscosum Vent. belonging to group of species with corolla irregularly salver-shaped, 3/4 in. long or less; and distinguished by calyx much enlarged in fruit and turning red, calyx deeply divided to the base, leaves cordate and tomentose beneath and simple flowers, from *Clerodendrum serratum* (L.) Moon. and *(Clerodendrum multiflorum* (Burm. f.) Kuntze syn. *C. phlomidis* Linn. f. alongwith other relevant species.

Genus *Clerodendrum* Linn. Species 70, in the warmer regions of both Hemispheres, chiefly in the Eastern; or species 100 nearly, mainly in the warm regions of Old World, a few in Tropical America. Salient features of the genus: Tree or shrubs, sometimes sarmerose. Leaves opposite, rarely 3-4-nate, simple, entire or lobed. Flowers in axillary cymes or terminal panicles, often leafy below, bracts conspicuous or small. Calyx campanulate; limb truncate 5-toothed or almost 5-partite, persistent, often accrescent, sometimes coloured. Corolla-tube slender, usually long, limb more or less oblique, lobes 5, spreading; stamens didynamous; ovary imperfectly 4-celled; stigma shortly bifid. Fruit a globose usually succulent drupe, 4-grooved and separating into 4 pyrenes including 1-3 sometimes suppressed. Seeds oblong. The leaves, roots, sprouts, flowers and other parts are medicinally useful of the plant *Clerodendrum viscosum* Vent.

The leaves and roots are applied externally over tumours and some skin diseases. Leaves are substitute for chiretta as tonic and antiperiodic medicine. Fresh leaves juice is useful as vermifuge and as bitter tonic and febrifuge in malaria which is specially useful in children. Leaves and flowers are useful in scropion-sting. Sprouts are considered useful in snake-bite.

Leaves contain bitter substance clerodin, proteinase and peptidase. Besides the active principle clerodin, the roots with hot petroleum and benzene yield and B-sitosteol successively.

Expressed juice of leaves is laxative, cholagogue and anthelmintic. Leaves are useful as vermifuge particularly in round worms infestation. Roots are also useful in colic. Leaves having a very disagreable odour are useful as bitter tonic, febrifuge or antipyretic, and also after attacks of ague and in worms ailments.

The plant is useful in veterinary medicine. Leaves or roots paste and juice are applied over ulcers with worms and skin affections like scabies or severe itchy affection in dogs and other animals or stocks. The plant is also used in ulcers, wounds and chronic ulcerations in animals.

Leaves powder is useful in worms, infantile malaria and as tonic, and roots powder or decoction in skin diseases. Leaves juice is given in worms. Bark is medicinally useful.

Roots are useful in bodyacho, dysentery, fits, convulsions, gastric desorders, chest pain, chest troubles, lungs affecttions, rheumatism and fever. Leaves are used in fever, malaria, remittent febrile conditions, headache, constipation, abnormal hairs falling and general debility.

Leaves are also useful as edible items in the form of drinks and vegetables.

Genus *Clerodendrum* Linn. is medicinally important as its various species are used in medicine alongwith other chemical, pharmacological and clinical importance, and a few also as ornamental or hedge plant.

Bhārangī or Bhārgī, the source plant *Clerodendrum serratum* (Linn.) Moon.; and Brahmayaṣṭī, *Clerodendrum indicum* (Linn.) Kutze.

Agnimantha or Araṇī, the source plant *Clerodendurm multiflorum* (Burm. f.) Kunzte., *Clerodendrum phlomidis* L.f.

Some species of *Clerodendrum* substitues, aduletrants or allied sources for both drugs of major place in indigenous medicine.

Clerodendrum inerme (Linn.) Gaertn. and *C. gragrans* Vent. are medicinally useful, and latter is of ornamental value.

Bhāṇḍīra or Bhaṇṭāka the Sanskrit name for the plant drug *Clerodendron viscsum* Vent. syn. *Clerodendron infortunatum* Gaertn.

Some other relevant species of the genus *Clerodendrum* Linn. as few are not referred above, and medicinally useful:-

Clerodendrum kaempferi (Jacq.) Sieb.

Velkameria kaempferi Jacq.

Clerodendrum squanmaṭtum Vahl.

Clerodendrum japonicum (Thunb.) Sweet.

Clerodendrum philiprinum Sehauer.

Volkameria japonica Jacq.

V. fragrans Vent.

Clerodendrum fragrans Hert.

C. fragrans Willd.

C. japonicum (Thunb.) Sweet var. *pleniflorum* (Sch.) Mah.

Clerodendrum wallichii Merrill.

Clerodendrum nutans D.Don.

Clerodendrum indicum (L.) O. Kuntze.

Siphonanthus indica L.

Clerodendrum siphonanthus R. Br.

Clerodendrum colobrookianum Walp.

7

Cochleospermum religiosum (L.) Alston

Bombax religiosum L.

Cochleopsermum gessypium DC.

Family: Cohleospermaceae (Bixineae)

Regional names: Gabdi, Kumbhi, Kumbi, Pillikapas, (Hindi), Ganglay, Sing (Marathi), Tanakhu (Tamil), Katira (Arabic), Appa kutakha (Malayalayam), Kendagogu (Telgu), Katira (Urdu), Tanukupututti, (Telgu), Ganeri, Gadhvi (Marathi), Kadhayo Gundar (Gujarati), Genjra, Arlu (Hindi), Gong, Gengal

Small naked tree, soft-wooded small tree with shrot thick spreading branches, the younger pens tomontose and bearing the scars of fallen-leaves and fruit-stalks, branchlets tomentose in deciduous trees. Leaves 3-8 in. diam. old glabrous, on slender petiole, 3-5 palmately-lobed, tomentose beneath, lobes acute or acuminate, entire, cordate at base, 7-nerved. Flowers 4-5 in. diam, in few-flowered terminal panicles, golden yellow, sepals silky, sepals unequal, silky, broadly oval, petals obovate, notched; fls. upto 8 cm. bread, petals golden yellow; anthers linear, falcate. Capsules 2-3 in. oval, 5-lobed, obvoid, cap. upto 10x8 cm., with reniform, brown and woolly seeds.

Flowering and fruiting: January- March; February-April or before the leaves appear (usually leafless in December-April) and fruits ripening during June-July or rains (summers or pre-monsoontime).

Distribution: Dry hills, Bundelkhand, Bihar, North Oudh, Orissa, Deecan, Siwalik range, Upper Gangetic Plains, Central India, Madhya Bharat, Southern India, Western Peninsula, Karnataka, Madras; generally in the decidous forests and hilly tracts and Siwaliks in Uttar Pradesh and dry hills; and also planted. Commonly in dry forests, particularly on stony hills in southern region, Madras and Tamilnadu state.

Genus *Cochleospermum* Kunth. with about 11 species all tropical in family Cochlespermaceae (initially in family Bixineae) and distinguishable by capsule almost 3-5 celled and leaves compound primarily (in tribe Bixeae) from *Bixa* Linn. having capsule 2-valved and leaves simple primarily. The group Bixeae has certain common characters such as petals broad, connected, without a scale or basal appendage and with anthers bursting by pores or short slits, showing similarity in species.

Genus *Cochleopsermum* Kunth. with salient features: Leaf blade palmately lobed, usually glaucous tomentose below. Flowers large, yellow showy; petals usually emarginate; disc none; filaments shortly connate at base; anthers linear; ovary 1-locular or incompletely 3-5-locular; ovules many, om 3-5-6 placentas. Capsules 3-5-valved, endocarp membranous, terete, smooth. Seeds covered by cottony hairs, cochleate, woolly, testa hard, embryo curved, seeds covered with cotton.

Cochleepsermum gossypium DC. is very showy tree in hot season blooming with bright yellow flowers of ornamentally golden colour in forests after the tree became leafless practically. Woods of tree very soft, light and spongy. Tree stands conspieuous for its shining flowers, habit and habitat alongwith particular features of various parts.

Small deciduous tree with short branches and deeply cracked thick bark, Leaves palmately 5-lobed, 4-6 in. diam.; lobes acuminate, more or less tomentose beneath; petioles thick, 6-9 in. long. Flowers 2-sexual, 3-4 in., across, in terminal panicles, appearing before the leaves; peduncle and pedicles covered with grey tomentum. Sepals 5, ovate or elliptie. 5 in. long, with numerous fine parallel veins. Stamens numerous, inserted on a disk; filaments. 5-7 in. long, filiform; anthers opening by a silt at the top or by a pore. Fruits pyriform capsule, 5- valved; valves 2-3 in. long. Seeds kidney-shaped,. 2 in. long, covered with soft silky wool.

Tree leafless in December or winters during the period from December to April). Common on dry slopes of the Outer Siwaliks, Upper Gangetic Plains. Plant found in flowering in March or April and fruiting in June or July.

Three main genera in family Bixaceae (later in Chocleospermaceae, Flacourtiaceae and others) may be distinguished on the basis of specific characters of leaves, flowers and fruits. Primarily the leaves are lobed, petals large and fruit a capsule in genus *Cochleospermaceae* Kunth.; but leaves are not lobed and petals none in other two genera when indehiscent fruits are in both of the genera; and they are differentiated of styles number which is 2 or more in *Flacourtia* Comm. while style only one in the genus *Xylosma* Forster.

The gum, leaves, flowers and bark of the plant *Cochleospermum religiosum* (Linn.) Alston. are medicinally useful.

The gums are sweetish, cooling, sedative and used in cough and gonorrhoea. Dried leaves and flowers are stimulant.

Tree yields a gum which is white and exuded from bark, and used in medicine. Gum is popularly named Katira. Gum of the plant is fried and useful in females specially indicated in backache, prolapse of uterus, leucorrhoea or menorrhagia, nervine debility,and joints pain similar complaints. Its internal use in female patients also helps to strengthen lungs and other organs by allevating cough, asthma and lungs and respiratory affections. It may be given about 1-3 gm, with warm water, milk or suitable vehicle.

Gums are useful in respiratory system disorders specially tuberculosis, cough, chronic cough, asthmatic troubles and other lungs diseases. A recipe is prepared by mixing Vamsalocana and Pippali *(Pipper longum)* with the gum and finelly powdering the drugs. this powders is given with honey once or twice a day about 1-3 gm.

The powder or decoction of bark is useful in jaundice. Roots powder or decoction is given in urinary disorders. The seeds are fried and given orally. Flowers and fruits are also edible. Plant is also useful in sores, tubercle glands and fistula. The gums are medicinally potent alike gum Tragacanth or it may be substitute by gum Katira exuded from the bark of plant.

Plant is also considered as anticancer ad hypotesnive drug. The bark is applied over fracture of bones in animals. Flowers are esteemed in offerings also. Seeds oil is edible.

Medicinal properties and actions of the durg are Kaṣāya-Madhur Kaṭu rasa, Sita virya, Kaṭu vipāka; Vātapitta sāmaka; Sangrāhi, Balya, Kāsahara, Sandhānīya, Vraṇaropaṇa; and theraeutically useful in Kasa, Svasa, Ksaya, Urahksata, Vrana, Bhagandra, Uccaraktacaea, Karkatarbuds, Kamala-Pandu, Raktapradara, Katisuka, Daurbalya, Garhasayabhramsa, Upadamsa and other ailments.

Kaṭṭīra: Siddha Bhaisajya Manimala

Silky wool from seeds is collected and this yellow-coloured wool utilised as cotton in pillows and other beddings.

8

Corallocarpus epigeus C.B. Clarke

Corallocarpus epigeus C.B. Cl.

Bryonia epigeus Rottle., W. & A.

Aeschmandra epigeus Arn.

Family: Cucurbitaceae

Regional Names: Mirchiakand, Khirkand, Akasgaddah (Hindi).

Kararinai (Bombay), Akashgrounded Nagdenda (Telgu), Kollanhovakii Zhauna (Malayalam),

Climbing or prostrate herb. Leaves 2 in. diam, broadly suborbicular, 3-5 anlged or lobed, punctate, or scabrid with minute, hairs; lobes often lobulate, obtuse, margins sinuous; petiole 1/4 in. or around. Flowers greenish-yellow. Male peduncle 1.5 - 2 in. and female peducle 1/4-1/2 in. long. or more, stout. Fruit stalked, beaked, ellipsoid or ovoid, suddenly narrowed into beak, reddish when ripe. Seeds about 6, ellipsoid, turgid, smooth, margined. Roots turnip-shaped.

Plant found in the areas of Upper gangetic plains; Uttar Pradesh (Bundelkhand), Madhya Pradesh, Gujarat, Punjab, Deecan peninsula, India. Ceylon and other countries.

Genus *Corallocarpus* Welw. Species 15, chiefly in tropical Asia and Africa and one in Tropical America.

Corallocarpus genus with specific characters in group of stamens 3 (except a few members), female flowers solitary usually, ovules horizontal, anther-cells straight usually; the petiole with no stipule-like bract in the axil and the flowers small, monoecious, pale-yellow; and *Corallocarpus* specific characters include ovoid, rostrate, circumscise over the base.

Genus *Corallocarpus* with salient features in general-Climbing or prostrate herbs, scabrid or subtomentose; tendrils simple; leaves petioled, roundish-cordate, somewhat thick, entire lobed or palmate; flowers very small, monoecious, males in small corymb at the apex of long peduncle, females short-pedicelled or sub-sessile, solitary or clustered; berry ovoid, circumscise, near the base, usually rostrate; smooth or nearly so, little margined.

The roots of the plant *Corallocarpus epigeus* Benth. ex Hook. f. are medicinally useful.

Roots contain a bitter principle like bryonin.

Roots are aperient, alterative and use in chronic dysentery, syphilitic rheumatism, chronic mucous enteritis and snake bite. The tuberous roots are emetic, purgative, aleximarphic, expectorant, antidote to snake poison, anti-cough, hiccup and asthmatic, anti-inflammatory and cleaner of wounds, anthelmintic and, antipyretic and other medicinal actions. The roots are used in various forms in treating several ailments for its medicinal efficacy indicated.

Tubers of this plant are especially considered quite useful as an antidote to venomous poisons in snake-bite cases. Tuber is ground on hard surface (stone plates or alike) and it is orally given with water in snake-bitten person. This medicine effects vomiting and purgation by making purification and emitting out the poison, and it counters venomous affect as antidoe to poison. Other measures of snake bite are to be taken as usu.

In cough disorders, the root in low dose by rubbing or grinding with warm water or other vehicle is given for expectorant effect and relieving from troubling cough.

Similarly the root is used in low doses in various ailments such as chronic fever, cough affections, erruptions and worms.

The tuberous root makes poisonous effect in high doses and constant or frequent use internally.

Tubers are pounded and paste is applied over swellings or inflammatory ailments.

Medicinal properties and therapeutic indications of the drug-Tikta rasa, Usna virya, Katu Vipaka, Viṣagḥna, Vāmaka, Sothahara, Recaka, Kasahara, Svasahara, Jvaraghna, Krmighna and other actions.

Sukanāsā, Nahikanda and Kaṭunāhī (synonyms Nahikā, Sukākhyā, Sukahvaya terms incorporated): Susruta Saṁhitā (Sutra. 42-18, Cikitsa. 1-114, 17-37), Astāṅga Hṛdaya (Uttar. 34-28, 35-47); Nahikā Astānga Hṛdaya (Uttar. 30-18)., and Soḍhala Nighaṇṭu.

Two kinds of Nahi-Tikta and Madhura (Sodhalạ).

9

Craterostigma plantagineum (Benth.) Hochst.

Torenia plantaginea Benth.
Family: Scrophulariaceae
Regional name: Baisurai (Hindi)

Perennial herb, densely pilose, acaulescent, with a thick stout root-stock, 1.3 cm. long, densely covered with several stout roots, 3-10 cm. long. Leaves radical, rosulate, 3-9 in a whorl, vertical, evate to ovate-lanceolate, sometimes spathulate, somewhat fleshy, 2.8-4 x 1.5-2.2 cm., entire, ciliate-margined, obtuse, glabrus or sparingly prominent beneath, base narrowed into a short-winged petiole; petioles 8-15 x 3.5 mm., pilose on both sides. Scape usually 2.5 to 10 cm. long, unbranched, solitary or more, arising from the centre of the leaf-rosette, quadrangular, pilose. Flowers violet purple, 1.5-2 cm. in length, usually paired sometimes more, in racemes. Bracts opposite, foliar, ovate-lanceolate-to lanceolate, concave, 8-15x 4-8 mm., sessile, entire, ciliate, acute, glabrous above, pilose on the back, with a prominent mid-rib, each enclosing one or more flowers. Pedicels 2-4 mm. long., lower pedicles forming corymbose racemes. Calyx tubular, 5-angled or ribbed, 6-8 mm. long, accesent, teeth 5, subequal, 1-2 mm. long in flower. and reaching upto 4 mm. in fruit. Corolla violet-purple, 1.2-2 cm. bilipped, upper lip erect, 2-1 lobed, 4-5 mm. lower lip 3-lobed, middle one lobe largest; corolla-tube 7-10 mm. long, slightly pubescent outside. Stamens 4, didynamous, anthers dimorphic; posterior pairs subincluded inserted in the middle of corolla tube; filaments filiform; anthers oblong-linear, glabrous; antetior pairs (stamens) exerted, filaments elongate, anthers gibbous. Carpels 2, syncarpous, placentation axile; ovaries oblong, ovoid or ellispoid, glabrous; styles filiform, dilated upwards, stigmas shortly bilamellate at the apex. Capsules oval or oblong, narrowed at the ends. slightly 5-angled, 8-1 x 0.3 mm., equal to calyx, smooth, glabrous septicidal, turning blackish when natured; valves 2, entire, style base petsistent. Seeds many, oblong, about 1x1 mm., flat, smooth on the lower surface, upper surface convex, tubercular-rugulose, brown.

Flowering and fruiting: August-April

Plant found in Madhya Pradesh, India. The roots of *Craterostigma plantaginea* Hochst. are mainly medicinally useful. The internal use of plant drug is made in treatment of nervine complaints, joints pain and swelling of joints and similar ailments generally fall under groups of rheumatic disorders, rheumatoid arthritis and gout.

The roots of the small herb are crushed and boiled in water for preparing decoction. Normal process of making decoction of raw drugs requires mixing of water four times or parts (1 : 4 proportion) and the mixture (of drugs and water) is is boiled till its one part remains and then the boiled mixture is decanted or filtered. Certain modification and additions drug powder are also made wherever indicated, and the process decoction includes other indications also in accordance to drug, diseases and therapeusis.

The decoction of roots this plant is orally administered twice a day about 8-10 ml. which may be regulated and changed in view of acuteness of trouble, age and therapeutic requirement. The use of decoction of herbal drug is usually made as single medicine; but the course of treatment may follow use of other anti-rheumatic drugs of internal and external application if considered necessary, particularly allied sympotoms and diseases in patient.

This oral plant remedy is considered quite useful for its therapeutical effectiveness in swellings conditions indicated, as antirheumatic herbal agent.

The thick roots stocks of herb may be collected during the rainy seasons as the aerial parts (leaves and flowers) making the plant conspicous in this stage; and the root stocks of herb, fairly on exposed, gravelly and shallow soils in the areas of occurrence, are procured and dried in shade for storing properly.

Another plant used in the name of Baisurai and for the almost similar therapeutic utility specifically in rheumatism, arthritis and gout. Usual practice of using *Pluchea lanceoloata* Oliver & Hierm, popularly as Baisurai (Hindi), is botanical source for Rāsnā, the well known major durg in indigenous medicine. There are several plants sources and substitutes in different regions. Present plant *Craterostigma plantaginea* Hochst. stands entirely different from *Pluchea lanceolata* O. & H. morphologically.

Vātanirmūlikā, Bahumūlā, the Sanskrit names for the plant drug.

10

Elytraria acaulis (Linn. f.) Lindau

Elytraria acaulis Brem. var. *acaulis*

Justicia acaulis Linn. f.

Tubiflora acaulis Kuntze

Elytraria cremata Vahl. excl. syn. *E. lyrata* Vahl.

Family: Acanthaceae

Regional Names: Patharasaga, Sasamula (Hindi), Gudapasari, Patharchata, Homuli, Nilakadambu; Daṣmori (Bombay).

Herb, 0-2 in., woolly, Leaves 2-5 in., sometimes obtusely lobed, pubescent at least on the nerves beneath, sessile or narrowed into a petiole. Scapes several, 3-10 in., clothed with bract-like scales. Spikes 1/2-4 in., harsh. simple or branched; bracts 1/4 in., margins scarious, ciliate; bracteoles scarious ciliate. Calyx segments lanceolate, scariosus, ciliate, the broad one entire at the apex. Corolla 1/4-1/2 in., white or bluish. Anthers muticous at the base; rudiments of 2 barren stamens sometimes (at least) present. Capsule 1/4 in., rigid, valves branched, and the scape sometimes very tall (American species).

Flowering and fruiting: July-September or November.

Plant found in Madhya Pradesh, Central Provinces, and Uttar Pradesh.

Distribution: Deecan Peninsula and Ceylon, common southwards; extending north to Delhi, and to the Eastern Himalaya, Tropical and South Africa, tropical and North America.

Genus *Elytraria* Vahl. species 3-4, American, 1 widely spread in tropical Africa and Asia.

Genus *Elytraria* Vahl. Herbs, nearly stemless. Leaves alternate, crowded, subradical. Scapes cover by imbricated bracts; spikes close, rigid, simple or divided; bracts spirally imbricated, not opposite; bracteoles smaller than the bracts. Calyx segments unequal, the largest sometimes 2-fid. Corolla small, white or bluish; tube linear, limb 2-lipped; lobes 5, oblong, imbricate in bud. Stamens 2, perfect, attached in the corolla-throat; anthers elliptic, acute; cells 2, parallel, with or without a minute spur at the base. Style shortly 2-lobed; ovules 6-10 in. each cell, superimposed. Capsule ellipsoid, acute. Seeds minute, ovoid, point without retinacula.

Elytraria Michx. non. cons. having salient features of erect or prostrate, not climbing habit with scapigerous, stameless and radical leaves, distinguishes from other genera of the family Acanthaceae, and particularly co-member genera (in tribe Nelsotieae) on the basis of 4-partite calyx, 2 stamens and bracts rigid, imbricate.

Tubiflora Gmel. (under *Elytraria*). Stemless or nearly stemless herbs. Leaves subradical alternate. Flowers in close-rigid simple or divided spikes. Fruits capsule. Seeds minute. Genus *Tubiflora* in family Acanthaceae (species upwards of 2,000 in tropical and warm temperate regions) with distinguishing characterstics: bracts rigid, peduncle of spike-covered with alternate scales; calyx 4-partite and stamens 4 in herb with sub-radical leaves, and anhers; and differing from *Nelsonia* R. Br. for bracts herbaceous, spike sessile or if stalked the peduncle without scales.

Tubilfora acaulis O. Kuntze. Herb, stesm none or upto 2 in. long. Leaves 3-8 in., obovate or oblanceolate, obtuse or apiculate tapering into a hairy petiole, more or less crenate, nerves beneath pubescent. Scapes several, usually longer than the leaves, clothed with small rigid elliptic acuminate bract-like scales. Spikes hard, simple or branched; bracts ovate, acuminate or spine tipped, hairy outside and with ciliate margins. Calyx segments pennicillate at the apex and with scarious ciliate margins, three of them narrowly lanceolate, the 4th. broader and sometimes 2-fid. Corolla pale blue or white. Anthers without basal spur. Fruit capsule. Plant flowering after the rainy season.

Upper Gangetic plains; Bundelkhand, Madhya bharat, Rohilkhand, Brijbhumi, Uttar Pradesh, Madhya Pradesh, Marwar. Southwards through the drier parts of Peninsular India and Ceylon, extending to tropical and south Africa and to tropical and north America.

Elytraria acaulis (Linn. f.) Lindau. Scapegerous, fibrous-rooted herb. Stems almost none. Leaves 23x9 cm., obovate, undulate, tapering below into a short, hairy petiole. Scapes many. usually longer or as long as the leaves. Spikes 2.5-8x 0.5x0.7 cm., simple or branched. Flowers white, pale-coloured, much exceeding the bracts. Bracts ovate, acuminate or spine-tipped. Capsules 6-8 mm. long.

Herb commonly growing on the ridges and adjacent hilly tracts in open places and shades of bushes, better in depressions and moist soils in shades. Delhi, Haryana and adjoining areas in northern region.

The roots, leaves and whole plant are chiefly medicinally useful of the plant *Elytraria acaulis* Lindau. Various herbal medicaments are of external and internal administration both in several kinds of ailments. Different complaints in human males, females and infants or children are covered through various medicinal uses of this plant drug. It is also useful in veterinary medicine.

Roots are procured after digging and cleaning well for making free from soils and other undesirable substances to make the drug material suitable for medicinal application. Roots are cut into pieces and then pounded by grinding for preparing the paste (lepa or malahara) for external administration in the form of paste, ointment or cream for the purpose of usage topically with or without bandages wherever necessary, and by following regular changes of paste, dressing and other routine measures during the course of treating with this herbal medicament of single drug.

The external application of this herbal paste prepared from roots of plant is useful for treatment of various ailments such as abscess, tumour, boils, inflammation, glandular oedema, burns, blisters, tissues hardening, nail discolouration, wounds or ulcers and other allied complaints; The specific application of this plant for external use over mammary glands inflammation, abscess and tumourous ailments particularly in females is important among these herbal uses of the paste in various complaints. Besides the use of roots in paste form, the root pieces are also usable by rubbing or grinding on a clean stone-slate or other hard base (like sandal) and then applied over the breasts in females suffering from inflammation, injury and abscess or any other similar ailining conditions. Thus bandage with paste or any adhesive and creamy application both are followed depending upon the stage, conditions in female patients and in other ailments commonly of all patients in general. In cases of mammary glands and other glands where the condition of hardening of tissues involved and cyst is developed or any tumourous growth formed, the external application of roots of this plant finds its useful remedial measure with effects to different extents and stages. In various ailments where paste is not to be applied or bandaged, the expressed juice (or by maceration or grinding) or roots and creamy receipe (by rubbing of root) in minor complaints is applied there.

Internal uses of the plant are mainly for fever, remittent type pyrexia, colis, diarrhoea, infantile disorders, throat horseness or throat affection, tonsil trouble and cold. In these ailments, the roots, leaves and whole plant are employed for making various medicinal recipes for using in treating them in patients of different age groups.

Whole plant specially leaves are boiled with some black pepper or marica *(Piper nigrum)* and infusion like tea is made and it is internally given about a cup or 8-10 ml. twice a day in case of fever particularly periodic types. Similar preparations with necessary changes suiting to needs of ailments, are useful in other complaints such as cold troubles of tonsil and throat, diarrhoea and other complaints to be treated through internal uses of this plant. The roots and whole plant specially leaves many also be dried up and fine powder is made of raw drug material, and the powder of plant drug is useful for internal administration 2-5 gms. with suitable adjutant and vehicle (anupāna) keeping the age, ailing condition and medicine need in view.

In cases of infantile complaints and specially rickets, marasmus and diarrhoea, the root piece is rubbed or mixed in mother's milk (breast feed) or in warm water, milk or any other suitable vehicle, one small teaspoonful medicine is given twice or thrice a day or 20 drops to 2 ml. depending upon the necessity and symptoms.

Juice of leaves after warming up slightly (tolerably) 3-6 drops are poured into ear in cases or earache. Infusion of whole plant is made and after filtering the liquid, it is useful 3 ml.-6 ml. for children of different ages for treating their cough ailments. Decoction of leaves is made after adding adequate water ad after it remains about 1/4 of liquid, the same is filtered or the infusion can also be prepared, the same is internally given 8-10 ml. twice a day in case of veneral diaseases.

The leaves, roots and whole plant are useful for preparing paste or applying after grinding well over the sores of animals and livestocks.

The plant material is procurable from shaded, moist place and on hilly slopes under the dense forests or as undergrowth the plants attaining luxurious growth and sometimes forming beautiful carpet type on grounds as its occurrence in open waste place is rather seldom. Practically the period ranging from rains till winters when the plant gets full maturity, is considered as suitable season for collection of roots and other parts of plant or whole plant alongwith flowers and fruits. The roots are developed by this time fully and goes suit long underground and the drug collectors are to dig out the roots from the areas of fair growth. In summer season, the collection of plant drug may become little difficult or scanty mainly due to absence of leaves or vegetative part of herb rendering the recognition of plant or its underground roots searchful as its typical radical leaves are easy indication for collection or deep roots and herb as a whole.

Sahasramūlā, Pādaprasarī, Mūlapatrā, Pāṣāṇasāka, Dīrghamulā and other Sanskrit names for *Elytraria acaulis* Lindau.

11

Enicostema hyssopifolium (Willd.) Verdoorn.

Exacum hyssopifolium Willd.

Enicostema littorale Bl.

Gentiana verticillata L.

Slevetia verticillata D.Don.

Exacum hyssopifolium Willd.

Ericoila verticillata Borkh.

Hippion orientale Dalz.

Cicendia hyssopifolia W. & A.

Adenema hyssopifolium G. Don.

Enicostema verticillatum (Linn.) Engl.

Family: Gentianaceae

Regional names: Chota-chirayata, Nahi, Nai, Kadvinahi (Hindi), Kadavinayi (Bombay), Vallari (Tamil-Malayalam).

Glabrous perennial herb, 4-20 in. high, branching from the base, erect or procumbent herb with 10-20 cm. height. Stems 4-20 in. terete or quandrangular, internodes short, erect or procumbent, usually 4-angled. Leaves sessile, decussate, 2.5-6 x 0.5-1 cm., ovate-lanceolate, small or sublinear, lvs. shape varying from linear to elliptic-lanceolate, 5-nerved, the two marginal ones often obscure. Flowers in whorled clusters, white, usually 3 in axils. Calyx 1/8 in. or around, lobes as long as the tube, obtuse with narrow membranous margins. Corolla-tube 1/8 in., lobes 1/10 in., elliptic, acute. Anthers included. Stigmas large, bilobed. Capsule about 4x4 mm., narrowed towards the base. Seeds small or minute, brown, foveolate.

Flowering and fruiting: June-September or rainy season

Distribution: Throughout India upto 1600 ft. alt. about, from the Punjab and Gangetic Plains to Ceylon, frequently near the sea or coastal region. Commonly in greater part of India; Ceylon and extending upto Java, Tropical and South Africa and the West Indies.

Occurring commonly in wet places; also found scatteredly in small patches stony grounds, along river banks and streams, bundhs and similar places in country.

Enicostema Bl. nom. cons. among terrestrial herbs jwith specific characters of flowers white, in sessile and axillary clusters.

Genus *Enicostema* Blume. Species 4, two in Tropical Africa including one species also in India, one in Madagascar and another in Tropical America. Salient features of the genus *Enicostema* Blume. Erect or decumbent branching herbs. Leaves opposite, sessile. Flowers small, in sessile axillary clusters. Clayx-tubes campanulate, tubes 5, lobes 8, lanceolate. Corolla tubular below, narrowly funnel-shaped above, lobes 5, small. Stamens 5, attached to the sessile-tube; filaments linear, with a small double-hooded scale on the inner side of each at the base; anthers erect, not twisted, acute. Ovary 1-celled, placenta slightly intruded; style short, stigma capitate, ovules many. Capsule ellipsoid. Seeds many, subglobose, faveolate or reticulated.

Genus *Enicostema* Blume. in family Gentianaceae (species 520 throughout the world, more abundant in mountainous regions); and the tribe II Chironieae having genera of leaves opposite, corolla-tube twisted to the right, ovary 1-celled and style filiform; and the genus *Enicostema* Blume distinguished by flowers regular in axillary clusters, from other relevant genera *Erythrea* Rich., *Canscora* Lamk. and *Hoppea* Willd. with different characters.

The leaves and whole plant *Enicostema littorale* Blume are medicinally useful.

The phytochemical and pharmacological screening of whole plant alongwith isolation of alkaloids and their effects provide information abouts chemical profile and pharmacological efficacy. An alkaloid gentianine previously isolated from the plant has been found to be an artifact. Its precursor has been identified as swertiamrin. Extraction of the plant with methanol and chromatography of the extract over akumina gave amorohous bitter substance. Aceytylation of this compound gave a crystalline acetate. The N.M.R. of the compound was found identifical with the NMR spectrum of swertiamrin tetracetate. The identity was confirmed by direct comparison with authentic sample. The infra-red spectra of the two samples were also identical. It contains bitter principle found in the plant. Plant contains bitter glycoside and opholic acid.

Plant is bitter, stomachic, tonic, laxative, Powder of whole plant is given with honey as a blood purifier and internally used in dropsy, rheumatism, abdominal ulcer, hernia, rheumatism, swellings, itches and insect poisoning.

The whole plant powder or decoction is given in skin diseases and periodic fever., and also as carminative and anti-inflammatory medicine.

The expressed juice, powder or decoction is quite effective in diabetes. It is useful in snake bite cases as an antidote of poison and antimalarial or antiperiodic herb. Whole plant is useful in veneral diseases.

Māmajjaka and Katunāhī, the Sanskrit names for the plant *Enicostema hyssopifolium* (Willd.) Verd. syn. *Enicostema littorale* Bl.

12

Orthosiphon pallidus Royle ex Benth

Family: Lamiaceae (Labiateae)

Regional names: Damanjri, Ajgur, Nagandha bavari, Dimenjar (Hindi). Low diffuse undershrub, 6-12 in. high; branches many from a woody root-stock, 4-angular, finely pubescent or sub-glabrema. Leaves petioled, not scented, ovate, obtuse or acute, coarsely serrate or crenate, glabrous or sparingly hairy, base cuneate, entire, petioled. Racemes rather short, whorls distant, 6-flowered; bracts minute, hairy; pedicels almost as long as the calyx in flower, hairy. Calyx enlarging to twice so long in fruit, hairy below; upper lip with 3 oblique lobes, lower lip membraneous, strongly parallel-nerved, the two central teeth narrowly lanceolate and ending in a long up-curved awn exceeding the upper lip; lateral teeth broadly lanceolate and with about straight awns; corolla white or lilac, 1/4 in. long, tube about as long as the calyx, upper lip shorter than the rounded and concave lower lip. Nutlets subglobose, smooth, pale-brown.

Flowering and fruiting: July-September or November

Throughout the greater part of India from Kashmir and Punjab to western Bihar and southwards to Travancore, extending to Gilgit, Baluchistan, Aden and Africa. Plant found in Sub-Himalayan tracts of North Oudh, the banks of Jamuna, Madhya Pradesh, Uttar Pradesh and provinces in India.

Genus *Orthosiphon* Benth.- Species about 50, in the warmer regions of the Old World.

Salient features of genus *Orthosiphon* with undershrubs or shrubs; flowers racemose in 6-or fewer-flowered whorls, bracts small; calyx tubular or campanulate, ovoid, deflexed in fruit; upper lip broad, lower lip 4-lobed, later lobes aristate, middle tubes subulate; corolla bilipped, tube often slender, straight or curved, tube as long as or exerted firm calyx tube, upper lip 3-4 lobed, lower lip entire, concave; stamens declinate, exerted, didynamous, filaments free; teethless at the base; anther cells confluent; stigma capitate, entire or marginate. disk usually gibbous; ovary 4-partite, style with a minute stigma; nutlets dry, ovoid or globose, smooth or nearly smooth with basal small scar.

Orthosiphon spiralis (Lour.) Merrill

Orthosiphon aristatus (Bl.) Miq.

Ocimum aristatum Bl.

Clerodendron spicatum Thunb. (non *O. spicatun* Benth.)

Orthosiphon stamineus Benth.

O. grandiflorus Bedding.

Ocimum grandiflorum Blume.

Ocimum longiflorum Ham.

Family: Lamiaceae (Labiatae)

Regional Names: Java Tea, Kidney-Tea Plant (English) twice as long as the corolla.

Plant stems 1-3 ft., 4-angled. Leaves in distinct pairs, 2-4 in., narrowed into the petiole. Racemes very lax-fid. Calyx 1/4 in. Corolla 1 in. glabrous, white or purplish. Nutlets broadly oblong, compressed, rugulose.

Distribution: Malaya, Philippine Islands, Australia, India, Burma, Martabin.

Plant occurring in Assam, Deccan Peninsula, Ana amallay Hills, Nicobar Islands; found in Manipur, Naga and Loshai Hills, Chota Nagpur, Western Ghats and Nicobar Islands.

Herb erect, slender and angled stem of *Orthosiphon spiralis* (Lour.) Merrill. with acuminate, ovate and coarsely toothed leaves, flowers white or purplish, in lax-flowered racemes, and nutlets broadly oblong, compressed and rugulose. The species belongs to the group of plants under genus with calyx-throat naked and stamens for exerted; whereas the calyx-throat naked and stamens included in *Orthosiphom pallidus* Royle. Some authorities find the taxon *Orthosiphon rubicundus* (D. Don.) Bentham. with included stamens.

Various species of *Orthosiphon* Benth. distinguishable in the genus *Orthosiphon* Benth. with salient characters and specifically calyx unequally dentate or 2-lipped and stigma entire; and leaves sessile in other species of the kind, but and rarely petioled in *Orthosiphon rubicundus* Benth. when the leaves petioled in other species such as *Orthosiphon diffusus* Benth., *O. pallidus* Royle, *O. incurvus* and other species.

Orthosiphon incurvus Benth.

Family: Lamiaceae (Labiatae)

Hairy usually sparingly branched undershrub with 4-angled stems, and with whorls of pale pink to mauve flowers in terminal interrupted spike-like clusters, Corolla c. 1.5 cm. with a straight or curved tube and with a 3-4 lobed upper lip and an entire lower lip. Calyx c. 8 mm., bell-shaped 2-lipped, the upper lip broad papery, the lower with 2 awned teeth and longer curved basal lobes; bracts tiny, ovate. Leaves 8-15 cm., ovate to ovate-lanceolate, coarsley toothed, narrowed to a short or long winged leaf-stalk; stems finely hairy., 15-90 cm.

Flowering and fruiting: February-November

Distribution: Central Nepal to Butan; 400-2000 m. alt. Forests, shrubberies; Godavari in Nepal.

Plant occurring in Subtropical Himalayas, Nepal, Sikkim, Khasia hills (about 3-4,000 ft. alt.); Eastern Himalaya.

Orthosiphon incurvus Benth. Puberulous, pubescent or tomentose herb, stem usually subsimple ascending 4-angled; leaves 3-6 in. petibled ovate or ovate-lanceolate coarsely crenate, bracts ovate, 2 lower calyx-teeth awned, corolla upto 1 in. straight or incurved, nutlets broadly ellipsoid, compressed asperulous. India, Nepal and Burma.

Orthosiphon incurvus Benth. Stem 1-3 ft., rarely branched. Leaves narrowed into winged petioles, rough or smooth above, sometimes of a fine purple beneath. Calyx in fruit 1/2 in., lateral teeth irregular, hardly awned. Corollas pale-pink, variable in size and curvature. *Orthosiphon rubicundus* Benth. consists to *O. incurvus* Benth., the other with more lanceolate subsessile leaves in the true *O. rubicundus* Benth. Among the species of *Orthosiphon* Benth., this species belongs to the group of plants with calyx-throat naked and stamens included in species having leaves petioled. The genus *Orthosiphon* Benth broadly falls among the plants of family Lamiaceae with creeping stems rooting at the nodes in general.

Othosiphon incurvus Benth. var, *elata.* Tall, branched, racemes densely tomentose, bracts large longer than the pedicels. A very large form with ovate-lanceolate leaves 4-7 in. long, scaberulous above and beneath. Corolla 1/2 in. long, tube slender. Eastern Nepal, Tambur and Khabili rivers (upto 6,000 ft. alt).

Orthosiphon rubicundus (D.Don.) Benth.

Plectranthas rubicundus D. Don.

(*Plectranthes rubicunda*)

Ocimum tuberosum Roxb.

Orthosiphon virgatus Benth.

Plectranthus mollissimus Wall.

Ocimum miris Ham.

Family: Lamiaceae (Labiatae)

Regional names: Jikipota (Mundari)

Erect, perenial herbs, with a woody, often tuberous rootstock. Stems 4-angled, glabrate or pubescent. Leaves sessile, ovate or ovate-lanceolate, combined into in interrupted, raceme-like inflorescence. Bracts minute. Calyx hairy; lower lip with 4 subulate teeth. Corolla white or pink. Nutlets suborbicular, compressed, punctulate.

Flowering and fruiting:	April-August; May-July
Distribution:	Western Subtropical Himalaya; from Central Nepal to Jammu (2,000-4,000 ft. alt.) and southwards to the Circars and Nilgiris. Upper Burma.

Plant occurring from Kashmir to Nepal and in Bihar, Uttar Pradesh West Bengal, Orrissa, North Circars, Deccan and western ghats (ascending upto 1,800 m. in hills).

Orthosiphon rubicundus Benth.

An erect much-Branched pernnial herb. 1-2 ft. high with a woody rootstock, the root often furnished with fusiform root-tubers. Leaves opposite, 2-4 in. long by 1-1.5 in. broad. sessile or shortly petioled, elliptic-oblong or oblanceolate, obtuse, coarsely serrate-dentate, cuneate at the base, pubescent on both surfaces, especially on the nerves. Flowers white, lilac or rose, distant, 6-flowered whorls in terminal recemes 6 in. or more long. Corolla 2-lipped, 2-5 in. long, its tube twice as long as the calyx. Stamens 4.

Fairly common in Dehradun and the Siwaliks in Uttar Pradesh; Upper Gangetic Plains.

Orthosiphon rubicundus (D. Don.) Bentham. Pubescent herbs. Leaves ovate, cuneate, up to 8x6 cm., Raceme 12-15 cm. long; bracts 2-3 mm. long, pubescent. Calyx 5 mm. long; corolla white; tube upto 7 mm. long. Stamens slightly exerted from corolla tube. Frequent in scrub, Karnataka, India.

Orthosiphon rubicundus (D. Don.) Bentham.

Plectranthes rubicundus D. Don.

Orthosiphon virgatus Benth.

Ocimum tuberosum Roxb.

Regional Names: Bankikir, Jikipota

Erect perenial herb with a wooly often tuberocus root stock. Stems slender 1-2 feet high, 4-angled, pubescent or glabrate. Leaves usually sessile 2-4 in long, ovate or ovate lanceolate, coarsely crenate or serrate, base cuneate, Flowers in rather distant whorls, bracts minute; calyx hairy, lower lip with 4 subulate; corolla white or pink, tube twice as long as the calyx. Nutlets suborbicular, compressed, punctutate.

Western Himalaya from Kashmir to Nepal ascending to 5,000 ft. and from West Bengal to the Nilgiri hillz, extending to Upper Burma and China. Plant not uncommon in the Sub-Himalayan tracts from Dehradun and Siwalik range eastwards; and frequent in scrub, Karnataka in India, and also in Burma.

Flowering and fruiting: May-July or blooming in April-June. Two species of *Orthosiphon* mainly differ as corolla-tube about as long as the calyx in *Orthosiphon pallidus* and Corolla-tube twice as long as the calyx in *Orthosiphon rubicundus.* Salient features of the species :

O. pallidus Royle ex Benth. An erect, diffuse herb, 15 cm. or more tall. Leaves 3-7 x 1.3-3 cm., ovate, crenate, petiolate, glabrous, greenish-yellow. Flowers 9 x 4 mm., white in lax, erect, verticillasters, arranged in a raceme. Calyx enlarging in fruit, deflexed in fruit. Nutlets subglobose.

O. rubicundus (D. Don.) Benth. Pubescent herbs. Leaves ovate, cuneate, to 8 x 6 cm. Raceme 12-15 cm. long; bracts 2-3 mm. long, pubescent. Calyx 5 mm. long; corolla white; tube to 7 mm. long. Stamens slightly exerted from corolla tube (stamens included characterized by certain authorities about the taxon).

Orthosiphon aristatus Mig (Bl:)

Orthosiphon grandiflora Boldingh.

Orthosiphon stamineus Benth.

Ocimum aristatum Bl.

Clerodendron spicatum Thunb.

Plant occurs in Assam, Deccan and Anamalai.

Orthosiphon thymiflorus (Roth.) Sleeren.

Ocimum thymiflorum Roth.

Orthosiphon glabratus Benth.

O. viscosus Benth.

Endostemon viscosus (Roth.) Ashby.

Orthosiphon thymiflorus (Roth.) Sleeren.

Ocimum thymiflorum Roth.

Orthosiphon glabratus Benth.

Ocimum viscosum Roth.

Orthosiphon viscosus Benth.

Orthosiphon tomentosus Benth.

Orthosiphon tomentus us var. *glabrata* Hook. f.

Orthosiphon tømentosus var. *viscosa* Hook. f.

Orthosiphon thymiflorus var. *temontosus* Sleesen.

Orthosiphon tomentosus var. *viscosus* Sleesen

Endostemon viscosus (Roth.) Ashby.

Family: Lamiaceae (Labiatae)

Regional names: Kattu-thirthava (Malayalam)

Erect herb, tomentose, pubescent or glabrate, sometimes viscid; leaves petioled, ovate, base rounded, cuneate or cordate, racemes elongate, bracts ovate, 4-lower calyx teeth-awned, corolla from half as long to thrice as long as the calyx, tube subincurved, nutlets subglobose compressed pale brown nearly smooth.

Distribution: Deccan Peninsula, on the Ghats and, and from the Konkan southwards. Ceylon.

Plant occurring in Orissa, Gujarat, and southern India, ascending upto 1,000 m. alt. in hilly regions.

Most variable plant comprising certain varieties and forms such as var. *tomentosus* proper, var. *viscosa,* var. *rubiginosa,* var. *glabrata,* var. *parviflora* and others having characterstic and general features showing distinction and commonity, in different regions of occurrence.

Genus *Orthosiphon* Benth. in family Lamiaceae or Labiatae (species about 600, chiefly in north temperate regions, or about 180 genera with over 3,500 species of cosmopolitan distribution, with Mediterranean as the chief centre) belongs to tribe I Ocimoideae and subtribe Euocineae with specific characters of lower lip of corolla flat or nearly so; and the characters of deflexed fruiting calyx, often long corolla tube and entire stigma distinguishes the genus from other genera in this group of generic plants.

In India 64 genera with 180 species, chiefly in mountainous regions, in family carrying very little forest importance but containing many herbaceous plants of more importance in medicine, perfume and aromatic olants, being mostly aromatic herbs which include *Orthosiphon* species.

The whole plant and leaves are chief parts of the herb *Orthosiphon pallidus* Royle ex Benth. which are medicinally useful. Various uses of the plant are for internal administration. This herb is useful in treatment of some ailments mainly fevers and urinary disorders.

Whole plant is pounded and mixed with adequate water for preparing decoction or infusion, ordinarily like tea, and after decatation the liquid medicine about 10 ml. orally twice or thrice a day is given in cases of fever specially in remittent and malarial kind of fever and periodic febrile conditions. The receipe may also be added black pepper (kali miraca) and other ingridient like sugar and ginger (ardraka) needfully, and the preparation is taken with suitable changes in quantity, frequency and period in view of age, complaints, symptoms and allied ailments including cough, bodyache and allied troubles.

Herb is useful in treating urinary disorders. Whole plant is macerated well in water or made infusion. This liquid duly decanted about 10 ml. is given twice in a day or depending on the needs and symptems in cases of troubles specially with burning sensation in micturition and scanty urine, and allied complaints of retention of urine generally. The quantity and period of use may change in suitability to ailing conditions.

Interestingly it is also believed sometimes, probably as saying, that the snakes when they become lesser poisonous or non-poisonous after casting off their slough (kencula) or papery skin, and then they used to swollow this herb in natural way, and the snakes gets vigour, strength and even poisonousness, by restoring the normal vigour. This is another indication or symbolic appreciation of medicinal potentiality of herb of its kind subject to extents of fact.

The plant in common or scattered in open grounds in certain areas of occurrence in various areas of distributional ranges. Generally the collection of herb is suitable during the period commencing from July-August or rainy season ending to October-November or winters out set when the plants flourish and flowering and fruiting over rendering the plant fully matured and medicinally quite potential. Fresh leaves and herb are also useful to collect and utilise in medicine whenever the same is available for medicinal utility and requirement.

Orthosiphon spiralis (Lour.) Merrill. is medicinally useful plants specially its leaves which are much valued in medicine and as therapeutically potent drug.

Leaves are made into infusion in the form of tea and one teacupful or half is taken twice a day. It is also called Java Tea due to its medicinal, common and mode of uses in particular region. The praparation may also be added other suitable ingredients and taken in about 8-10 ml. twice or thrice depending on the age, symptoms and medicinal necessity. This kind of preparation is useful in complaints of urinary system as remedy for kidney and urinary bladder disorders. For this medicinal purpose, fresh leaves are quite potent and dried or leaves plucked a few days back (and stored properly) are also employed for preparing the infusion indicated for medicinal application as the herbal foliage mainly entire into therapeusis.

This drug occurs in commerce as small, oval finely toothed leaves, rolled up like tea. It is almost odourless and tasteless. It is reported to be official in a number of pharmacopoeias. The standard drug is prescribed to contain moisture 13% ash 8% and water soluble extract 30% the best grades yield 40-45% water soluble extract..

The chemical constituents of the plant find that the activity of leaves of herb is attributed mostly to the presence of high percentage (0.7-0.8) of potassium salts and a bitter glycoside, orthosiphonin. The leaves are reported to contain also a saponin, an alkaloid, an essential oil (0.2-0.6%), tannins, organic acids particularly tartaric, citric and glycolic, urea and a greenish fatty oil.The saponin yields arabinose and glucose (or fructose) besides a sapogenin. The essential oil is yellow in colour and has a strong unpleasant odour. The unsaponifiable matter of the fatty oil contains sitosterol and a-amyrin. A process has been patented in Germany for the extraction of an active diuretic principle (m.p. 222-24^0) in a yield of 0.22% in the leaves.

The plant drug is highly cumulative diuretic, most useful in nephrosis and servere cases of oedema or dropsy. An infusion of leaves is given as a specific treatment of various kidney and bladder diseases including nephrocirrhosis and phosphaturia. It is also useful in rheumatism and gout. The use of medicine renders the urine clear and help to make it normal. This herbal medicine has the property to increase the alkalinity in blood or or making it alkaline normally; and thus usefully suggested in urinary affections.

The presence of orthosiphonin and potassium salts in the drug helps in keeping uric acid and urate salts in the solution, and thus prevents deposits (calculi and allied anomalies) from forming in the kidney. Leaf extracts lowers the blood sugar in diabetic patients but not consistently. It stimulates glycogen formation and exerts a sympathicolytic action. It is also used as a hypertensive agent.

The leaf drug had been in therapeutic use of South-east Asian region in begining as before the World War II, it was cultivated for its leaves mostly in Indonessia, and it was than taken up for cultivation to a small extent in South Vietnam. It can be grown on a wide range of climate and soil, but thrives best under thin shade. It can serve as a remunerative catch crop in coconut or rubber plantations. The plant can be grown from seeds or by cuttings. By raising from cuttings, it may give appreciable flush of leaves in 2-3 months from the time of planting. Flowers should be removed as and when they appear as they are supposed to deprive the leaves of their active constituents. The leaves are gathered in the same way as tea at intervals of 2-3 weeks, the tender bud and the shoots with 2-4 leaves being nipped off by hand. Leaves are then withered for c. 24 hours and dried in the oven or in hot air driers 1 kg. of green leaf yields about 0.17 kg. of cured leaves. When the leaves are crisp-dry, they are crushed and immediately sifted through a wire sieve with 3 mm. square meshes. The finished product is stored in air-tight tins or packed in tea chests ready for export. There was steady demand (during 1960s) for the drug in form of a tincture or in tablets. Sun dried products are preferred to oven dried, since it is considered that high temperature destroys the medicinal potency and adverse the properties existed in the drug substance.

Orthosiphon pallidus Reyle ex Benth. contains Orthosiphonol, the active principle, which was has been isolated and chemical study is carried out; and phytochemical screening has also isolated choline and betain from the plant.

Whole plant and leaves of *Orthosiphon thymiflorus* (Roth.) Sleeren are medicinally useful. Decoction of whole plant is prepared and decanted; and this preparation about 8-10 ml. is given twice in diarrhoea and piles. Infusion or decoction of leaves of plant is prepared and given about 8-10 ml. in cases of fever.

Leaves of *Orthosiphon thymiflorus* (Roth.) Sleeren syn. *O. glabratus* Benth. are also used in external application. The leaves are pounded and applied over cuts and wounds as they are considered to possess curative properties of wound or ulcer healing up.

Orthosiphon rubicundus Benth. is medicinally useful. The tubers of this plant are eaten and they yield a starch. There are considered as a remedy for colic.

In general, the medicinal properties and action of drug mainly are Kaṭu-Tikta rasa, Uṣṇa vīrya, Ruksa Tīkṣṇa guṇa, Kaphavāta Sāmaka, Mutrala, Jvaraghna, Sītaprasamana, Kāhaghna, Aṅgamerda prasamana, Vraṇaropaṇa, Pramehahara, Madhumehanāsana, Mutrāmayahara, Bastirogahara, Vṛkkarga hara, Hṛdya, Balya, Vātavyādhi and Āmavāta nāsaka, Mutrāsmarī-sarkarā pratibandhaka, Rucikāraka and other properties and actions and therapeutic indications.

Devamañjajrī, the Sanskrit name for *Orthosiphon pallidus* Royle ex Benth.

Another probable botanical source or substitute plant for Arjaka and its kind Sveta Kuṭheraka.

There kinds of Arjaka with specific synonyms or Sanskrit terms-Kutheraka (Kṣudrapatra, Arjaka, Kuṇṭha, Vaikuṇṭha), Kathinjara (Paramāsa, Bilvagandha, Svetaparṇa) and Vaṭapatra (Gandhapatra, Kapittharjaka) in Kaiyadeva Nighaṇṭu (Oṣadhi varga 1560-1562).

(a) Arjaka, Kuṭhera and Kuṭhoraka (Sveta Kuṭheraka): Caraka Saṁhitā (Sutra. 2-3, 27-99; Nidan. 2-2; Viman. 7-17, 22, 8-149, 158; Cikitsa. 3-266, 27-57; Kalpa. 1-28), Susruta Saṁhitā (Sutra. 38-18, 46-221), Aṣṭāṅga Hṛdaya (Sutra. 6-106; 10-31; Uttar. 22-74), Kaiyadeva Nighantu (oṣadhi varga, 1560-1562) and several works of indigenous medicine.

(b) Arjaka-Caraka Saṁhitā (Sutra. 14-31, 26-109, 27-167; Viman. 8-140; Srir. 8-54; Cikitsa. 7-111, 11-84, 12-65, 70, 37-54), Susruta Saṁhitā (Sutra. 38-48, 39-6, 46-221, 235; Cikitsa. 9-18; Uttar. 11-11, 39-267), Aṣṭāṅga Hṛdaya (Sutra. 6-106, 17-7; Cikitsa. 3-142, 6-19), Kaiyadeva Nighaṇṭu (osadhi varga, 1560-1562), Rāja Nighaṇṭu (Karvīrādi varga, 156-158), and several works of indigenous medicine.

Othosiphon pallidus Royle ex Benth.; and also *Orthosiphon grandiflorus* Boddingh. and *Orthosiphon glabaratus* Benth. as other probable substitutes, the source plants for Sveta Kuṭheraka Arjaka and Kaṭhiñjara-*Ocimum* sp.

13

Pentanema indicum (L.) Ling.

Inula indica L., *Inula indica* Willd.

Vicoa indica (L.) DC.

Vicoa auriculata Cass.

Deronicum calcaratub Roxb.

Family: Asteraceae (Compositae)

Regional Name: Banjhuri, Banasirsa (Hindi), Gurhmi, Palmadardu, Pottuchedi

Suffruitiscent herbs upto 1 m.; stem reddish-brown, serete, grooved, glabrous with age. Leaves upto 8x1.2 cm., ovate lanceolate, acute. cordate-hastate and amplexicaul below, entire, scabrid along margin, pubescent beneath. Heads 1.3-1.5 cm. across, usually solitary on long peduncles; bracts lanceolate, acute, hairy, the outer shorter. Ray florets about 22, ligule upto 0.5x6.2 cm., elliptic-oblong, 3-dentate, bright yellow. Disc florets many, yellow. Achene glabrous in female, hairy in bisexual; pappus scanty in bisexual, none in female.

Flowering and fruiting: April-November

Distribution: Central and Western Peninsular India, and Sri Lanka. Plant growing throughout the drier parts of India, from the Punjab to South India, Ceylon and also found in Burma.

Vicoa indica (Willd.) DC. An erect, branched, rigid herb. Leaves sessile, lanceolate or oblong-lanceolate; basal auricles round or hastate. Heads yellow bright yellow, 7-18

mm. in diam., heterogamous. Involucral bracts erect. Pappus of ray florets absent; of disc florets few, slender hairs.

Plant flowering ad fruiting during October to March; common on dry soil of fields and unsued grounds in Delhi, Haryana and Punjab, and neighbouring parts of region; the hotter parts of plains in northern India.

Inula indica Linn. A Slender rather rigid roughly pubescent often viscid herb. Stems 1-3 ft. high, the upper portion with many spreading branches. Leaves sessile, usually 1-2 in. long, but often scabrid on both surfaces; basal auricles rounded or hastate, sometimes laciniate. Heads on long slender spreading peduncles. Invol-bracts slender, scarcely recurved. Flowers orange-yellow; ligules revolute, as long as involucre. Achenes pale, terete, sparsely hairy. Pappus of ray-flowers O; of the disc few, slender, free at the base.

Plant growing in the Upper gangetic plains where common in most parts of the area. Distributed (upto lower heights) in the western Himalayas and throughout the drier parts of India; Central province and central India, and various provinces; Bihar, Uttar Pradesh, Madhya Pradesh and West Bengal and Tamilnadu, southern parts of country.

Vicoa auriculata Cass. A usually much branched slender rigid leafy herb, 1-3 ft., with spreading branches. Leaves 7 by 1.5 in. maximum and more commonly 1-2 in., base always rounded; auricles rounded or hastate, sometimes gashed. Hedas on long slender; ligulae revolute, as log as the involucre. Achenes pale, terete, sparsely hairy; pappus hairs few, slender, free at the base.

Throughout the drier parts of India, from Punjab to Burma and southwards, ascending the western Himalayan region (4,000 ft. alt.), and in Ceylon.

Genus *Vicoa* Cassini. Annual or perenial herbs. Leaves alternate, usually entire, pinnately veined, mostly amplexicaule at the base. Heads solitary, axillary or leaf-opposed, peduncled, usually radiate, rarely discoid; involucral bracts multi-seriate, narrow-acuminate; receptacles sometimes raised, glabrous. Outer florets few, female; the corolla ligulate, 2-dentate; the outer ligules broad, 2-3 dentate, the inner terete and subulate. Anthers sagitate below. Achenes angled, not ribbed, glabrous or hairy; pappus 1-seraite, smooth, scanty or none.

Vicoa Cass. genus of larger family Compositae (co-extensive with dicotyledonous vegetation with genera about 1,000 and species about 8,000) in Tribe Inuleae differing from Astereae in anthers tailed (except *Laggera* Sch.) having heads heterogamous and heads rayed, and differs by *Pulicaria* Gaertn. with pappus double rowed and ocuterscaly whereas *Vicoa* with pappus in a single row, scanty or absent. Genus *Vicoa* with 6 species in tropical and western Asia and Africa.

Pentanema vestitum (Wall. ex. DC.) Ling

Vicoa vestita Benth.

Pentanema radiatum Boiss.

Inula vestita Wall.

Vicoa vestita (Wall. ex DC.) Benth.

An erect, woolly, faintly scented herb. Stems reddish. Leaves oblong or linear-oblong, broadly auriculate, 5-10x1-2.5 cm. Heads bright yellow, about 0.7x2 cm., corymbose, heterogamous, radiate. Achenee oblong-cylndric, sparsely hairy.

Plant flowering and fruiting during February to March, spring season or around. A woolly and softly hairy herb; with leaves oblong or linear-oblong or obtuse or subacute from a broad auricled base serrate, involucre bracts squarrose lips filiform recurved, and achenes subsilky. Drier parts of India from Marri, and the Punjab to Scind, Patna, Bihar and the Konkan, Sikkim; Western Tibet, at Iskardo. Distributed in Afghanistan. Herb found in waste places and along Jamuna banks in Khadar area on moist soils, also on unused grounds, often becoming gregarious (near garden lands and other similar places), in Delhi, Haryana and adjoining parts of region.

Inula vestita Wall. syn. *Vicoa vestita* Benth. A. softly hairy or woolly herb, 10-18 in. high. Leaves 1-2 in. long, oblong or linear from a broadly auricled base, obtuse or subacute, serrate, thin. Involucre-bracts squarrose, the tips filiform, recurved. Heads bright-yellow, 2.4-1 in. across; ligules long, narrow, spreading. Achenes slightly silky, small. Plant growing in the Siwalik ranges and in Sub-Himalayan tracts of Rohilkhand and North Oudh, in the upper gangetic plains and adjacent regions.

Two species of *Vicoa* Cass. differ as *Vicoa vestita* Benth. ex Hook. being erect, woolly herbs with involucral bracts of recurved tips, whereas *Vicoa indica* (Willd.) DC. having erect, rigid herbs with involucral bracts erect. Both herbs, former villous and later viscid or glabrate; and as such *vestita* shorter and stouter plant than preceding and with more numerous and narrawer ligules; though achenes and pappis similar in both species having a similarity. Other species of *Inula* Linn. particularly two (*Inula cappa* DC. and *Inula rubicaulis* Clarke. earlier grouped) shrub in comparison with distinct characters, and descriptions.

Another species *Vicoa cernus* Dalz. occurring in the hills of Konkan and Western Deccan. Annual, selnder, sparsely pubescent, lower leaves sortlt petioled elliptic acuminate serrate, upper sessile contracted to a small auricled base, invol.-bracts squarrose tips filiform recurved. Herb rather slender, very similar in habit to *Vicoa auriculata* Cass., but differing in the leaves and involucre bracts. Herb also in

Upper gangetic plains; Flowering and fruiting during summers or hot months. Karnataka province, Belgaum. *Vicoa vestita* Benth. shorter and stouter than *Vicoa cernua* Dalz., but similar in achenes and pappus.

The roots, leaves, whole plants, twigs and other parts of the plant *Pentanema indicum* (L.) Ling. syn. *Vicoa auriculata* (Willd.) DC. are medicinally useful.

The roots are useful in birth control as antifertility drug. The twigs are abortifacient. Roots are used in tooth and gums affections; and useful in toothache and gingivitis.

Whole plant is useful in jaundice. Leaves and roots are useful in kidney disorders and urinary complaints, and also leaves in stomach troubles.

Medicinal properties and action of the durg Tikta-Kaṣāya rasa, Uṣṇa vīrya, Kaṭu vipāka; Laghu-usna guṇa; Vātakapha nāsaka, pittasamsamana; Garbhasrāvakara, Prajāniyamana, Dantya, Pittavirecaniya, Sūlaprasamana; Kandu-Kamala, Mutrāmaya-Vṛkka roga, Sirahsūla, Dantasūla, Dantamūlagata vikāra and other roga for therapeutic indications.

Internal and external mode of administration, in various forms of decoction, infusion powder, paste, juice and as other recipes and usage.

Parts used (upādeyāṅga) roots (mūla), leaves (patra), whole herb (pañcāṅga) and others (anya aṅga) including flowers (puṣpa) and twigs (sākhā).

Vandhyāvarī or Bandhyāvarī, the Sanskrit name for *Pentanema idicum* (L.) Ling. syn. *Vicoa auriculata* (Willd.) DC.

14

Rivea hypocrateriformis (Desr.) Choisy.

Convolvulus hypocrateriformis Desr.

Rivea hypocrateriformis Choisy.

Lettsomia bona-nox Roxb.

Argyrea uniflora Sweet.

Rivea fragrans Nimmo.

Convolvus candicans Wall.

Lettsomia uniflora Roxb.

Rivea ornata Aitch.

Argyrea bona-nox Sweet.

Family: Convolvulaceae

Regional Names:	Parh, Phang, Guwal-kakri, Kidura, Mustakeerai (Hindi)
English:	The 'Midnapore' or 'Clove-scented creeper'

Large climbing shrub. Stems of old plant often very stout, in climbing or spreading shrub of usually stout or tough stems with grey bark, thin; and young shoots milky-pubescent. Leaves 1.5-2.5 in. or 5-7 x 6-7.5 cm., rarely broader than long, orbicular, obtuse, emarginate, mucronati, usually broadly cordate at the base, glabrous or nearly so above, appressedly silky hairy beneath, with a pair of purplish glands at the base of lamina; basal nerves 5-7; petioles 1/2-2 in. long, with an obscure gland on each side of the apex. Flowers pure-white, clove scented, usually solitary being 1-flowered, axillary, peduncles short, sometimes 2-flowered; or more pedicels very short, in the axils of linear deciduous bracts; sepals 1/2 in. long, ovate-elliptic, obtuse, silky hairy; corolla 2.5-3 in. long, tube very long limb upto 2 in. across, glabrous or sparsely hairy outside. Fruit globose, about 1/2 in. diam., tipped with the persistent base of the style, brown, glabrous polished. Seeds 1-4 in berry.

Flowering and fruiting: August-November or around.

Western India; in dry forests from Lahore and Bihar to Mysore, common in Assam. Plains of Punjab, Rajputana and Sind to the Deccan, and from Assam and Bengal to South India. Often found within the area of Upper gangetic plains and the Siwaliks specially in the forest tracts of Merawara, Bundelkhand, Madhya Bharata and other parts of Madhya Pradesh and Uttar Pradesh; also in Delhi hilly tracts bordering Haryana and Punjab; Northern and Central India.

Rivea hypocrateriformis (Desr.) Choisy. also occurring in areas of Karnataka and Madras, Grey-tementose, climbing shrubs. Leaf reniform-ovate, cordate, shortly acuminate to 4 x 5 cm. Peduncle usually sub-terminal, 1-3-flowered; sepals oblong-lanceolate. obtuse, to 0.8 cm.; corolla white, to 5 cm. long. Fruits ovoid, brown, to 2 cm. long. Flowering in July.

Flowers of *Rivea hypocrateriformis* Choisy. fragrant, odoriferous or clove-scented. Pure white and clove-smelling flowers open at sunset and close, and wither the next morning; the flowers remain closed during the day. or sunlight; Flowers characterstics for hue and opening at sunset and closing at sunrise.

Genus *Rivea* Choisy-species about 10, three in India and the rest South American. Genus with climbing shrub; leaves cordate, more or less silky beneath, long-petioled, leaves simple with 2 glands at the tip of petiole. Cyme peduncled, 1-3-flowered, bracts narrow, short, 2-3 in number. Sepals ovate or lanceolate-oblong, subequal. Corolla large, white, salver-shaped, tube narrow, cylindric, limb with rounded plicate-lobes or limb shallowly lobed. Staminal filaments short, hairy toward the base or stamens included; pollens spinulose, anthers narrow, oblong, straight. Ovary 4-celled, or 4-locular, ovules 4, style filiform, ovule 1 per locule; stigmas 2, linear-oblong. Fruit subglobose, dry, indehiscent or opening irregularly, often 1-celled from the absorption of the sept, apiculate. Seeds 1-4, glabrous, surrounded by mealy pulp.

Mainly two species of *Rivea* genus in India. *Rivea hypocratteriformis* Choisy resembles with other species *Rivea ornata* Chois.

Rivea ornata Choisy.

omia ornata Roxb.

Convolvulus candicans Roth.

Argyrea ornata Sweet.

Rivea ornata var. *griffithii* Clarke.

Regional names: Phand (Marathi), Phanji, Baravata Muchuttai (Tamil), Boditige (Telgu),

Large spreading shrub or sometime shrub twiner. Branchlets stout, white-tomentose; stems subherbaceous, hardly ever twining. Leaves 3-6 in. long, usually broader than long, orbicular or reniform, obtuse, somewhat emarginate and often apiculate at the apex, rather silky beneath, lobes rounded; petiole shorter than the leaves, with a greeninsh gland on either side of the apex, petiole 1-2 in. long. Peduncles as long as the petioles, usually 7-flowered, bracts lanceolate or narrowly oblong, deciduous.

Deccan Peninsula, common in dry forests; and Ceylon, in the hotter parts of the Islanda. In India, the eastwards to North Bengal, and the Sikkim Terai; Central India, Upper gangetic plains, Siwalik ranges and other parts; Konkan, Deccan and Carnatic regions in country.

Flowers white, fragrant; sepals about 1/4 in. long, ovate lanceolate, acute, thick, silky-hairy outside, persistent;

corolla-tube 2-3 in. long, limb about 2-2.5 in. diam.; stigmas small. Fruits berry, oblong, pointed, 1-celled, globose, mucronate by the style base, yellow-brown, nearly dry. Seeds usually solitary.

Flowering and fruiting: August-November

Rivea ornata Chois. generally resembling with former species but the hair on the stems beneath the leaves and on the sepals is less copious, and much less white in regard to *Rivea hypocraterformis* Choisy, as essential distinction lies in the sepals which are smaller and more obtuse; thus the species are very nearly related and needy for difference.

Rivea genus in family Convolvulaceae with flowers solitary or in cymes and capsules valvular or operfular in regard to particularly several genera (e.g. *Cressa, Evolvulus, Rivea Argyrea* and others) but style 1 undivided in *Rivea* with fruits indehiscent, bacate, coriaceous or crustaceous, the flowers in white colour, salveform, stigmas linear-oblong differentiates it from flower characters of *Argyrea* on account of rosy or purple flowers in colour and funnel form in shape with globose stigmas. On the basis of fruits, the genus *Rivea* (in Tribe Convolvulaceae with corolla-tube plaited or induplicate in bud, initially in large family Convolvulaceae) the fruits indehiscent majorly in four genera and the genus *Rivea* serves distinction by stigmas 2 in linear-oblong shape from other of this group.

Genus *Argyrea* is closely allied with *Rivea* but differs for linear stigmas and dry or nearly dry fruit.

Mainly these two species of *Rivea* Choisy differs on the basis of flowers and leaves: *Ri hypocrateriformis* with sepals ovate, obtuse, peduncles usually 1-flowered; leaves rarely broader than long; but and *R. ornata* with sepals lanceolate, acute, peduncles usually by ovate-lanceolate or ovate-oblong and acute-calyx-segments, shorter peduncle and few-flowered cymes.

Rivea laotica Oeststr. closely allied to *R. ornata* (Roxb.) Choisy also rarely occurring in the Upper gangetic plains and Siwaliks, but distinguishable by longer peduncles, more-flowered cymes, oblong, obtuse outer calyx-segments and characterised by its erect herbaceous habit among other species of large woody climbers in case of all other members of genus *Rivea* Choisy.

Erect, perennial, suffruticose herb or undershrub with woody base and several stems from the base, simple or branched, terete or angular, densely appressed white hairy. Leaves orbicular eniform, with deeply cordate base, white margined, retuse, glabrous above, appressed white-pulescent on lower surface, with a pair of glands at apex of lower side of petiole Flowers white, 1-10-flowered cymes, axillary. Capsule with 4 seeds. Indo-China, India.

Rivea ornata Chois. whole plant is medicinally useful in an ointment for phthiriasis and in a preparation for piles. It is external application of plant. Young leaves and shoots of vegetative part are edible.

The roots are chiefly medicinal useful of the plant *Rivea hypocrateriformis* Choisy.; and the leaves, fruits and whole plant are medicinally utilised.

The roots are pounded and boiled in water to make the decoction and after the decantaion or filteration, this preparation about 8-10 ml. is regularly or at short intervals. This is administered in cases of snake-bite. Few margaosa leaves or nimba patra (*Azadirachta indica*) and Black pepper or marica (*Piper nigrum*) in the receipe also be added. A timely administration of the medicinal preparation may help to prevent development of signs of aspysia (popularly called 'gaṭā' or other names) under advancing stage in venomous snake causing severity. Other routine and first aid or emergent measure for treatment are also followed, and this oral medicament is one of the anti-venom herbal agents; and it also belongs to some important herbal drugs useful against snake-bite such as Gunishar, Parh, Kali gunishar and Parh, the popular names of certain medicinal plants which include the plant drug *Rivea hypocrateriformis* Choisy.

In hysteria, fits, giddiness and convulsions, the roots in form of decoction or powder about 8-10 ml. or 3-6 gm. are given to patients. Leaves powder or expressed juice about 2-4 gm. or 2-4 teaspoonful twice in a day are taken in condition of sexual weakness, spermatorrhoea, seminal affections and similar complaints.

Whole plant pounded and its paste or juice is applied over painful tooth and swollen gums. Fruits are edible and leaves (young leaves) or shoots are employed for preparing fried vegetable as medicated food item.

Source plant of this drug is extensive woody clomber in habit, commonly found on spiny bushes, small trees and particularly on hedges along roadsides and cultivated fields and other various places in the areas of occurrence. During rainy season, the collection of raw material, or drug is practically possible, and during the period ranging from rains to winters when the plants get full maturity after flowering and fruiting. After the digging up roots found very long, stouts and quite deeply underground, they are dried up in shade and kept in airtight containers for medicinal uses.

Phañjī: Caraka Saṁhitā (Sutra. 27-96), Susruta Saṁhitā (Sutra 38-14, 18; 46-249, 257; Kalpa. 1-61; Uttar. 40-113, Aṣṭāṅga Hṛdaya (Cikitsa. 9-24) and other works of indigenous medicine. Kaiyadeva Nighaṇṭu (Osadhi varga, 655/656).

Phañjī as the drug of independant existence as well as a synonym for Bhārgī and Brāhmaṇayaṣṭikā. Phanji and Padma (a variety of Bhargi source plant *Premna herbacea* Roxb.) co-synonymous; Phañjī sāka as vegetable. (Kaiyadeva Nighaṇṭu, Osadhi varga, 1134).

Medicinal properties and actions of Phañjī.

Kaṭu, Tikta, Kaṣāya rasa, Uṣṇa vīrya, Kaṭu vipāka, Rūkṣa-laghu guṇa, Pācana, Kaphavāta sāmaka, Rucikara, viṣṭambhī, Viṣṭabhi, Kāsaghna, Svāsahara, Svalpamalā, Balya, Dantya and other properties and therapeutic actions and indications.

15

Sauromatum venosum (Ait.) Kunth.

Sauromatum pedatum (Willd.) Schott.

Arum guttatum Wall.
Arum venosum W. Ait.
Arum sessiliflorum Roxb.

Sauromatum guttatum (Wall.) Schott.

(incl. var. venosum (W. Ait) Engler)

Family: Araceae

Regional names: Bhasmakand (Hindi), Loth (Bombay)

Genus *Sauromatum* Sochottin family Araceae distinguishable by some characters mainly plants with inflorescens preceeding that leaf and staminate flowers densely packed; leaf pedately 7-9 lobed and lower seathe margins fused into tube; which make difference from *Amorphophallus* Boume ex Deccaisne (nom. cons.) by its leaf ternately divided and dichotomously decomposed and lower spathe margins overlapping, as both genera have compound or deeply lobed; and another genera *Arisaema* Martius ma be separated by plants with inflorescens and leaves simultaneous and staminate flowers scattered, the three genera belonging to the ground or terrestrial plants with glabrous leaves.

Salient features of the genus *Sauromatum* Schott. Cormous, deciduous herbs. Leaf solitary, palmately deeply 7-9-lobed, venation reticulate; spathe shortly peduncled, entirely withering, but with margins connate in tube below and opening into long, narrow blade; spadix elongate, divided into 5 parts; pistillate, sterile area with clavate pistillodes, naked interstice, staminate portion, and elongate, naked appendix; stamens free, not grouped into flowers; ovules 1-2, basal.

Perennials, with a depressed-globose tuber. Leaves 1 or rarely 2, appear after flowers, on a 50-100 cm. long, purple blotched petiole, pedately partite; segments 3-10 (-15), elliptic-obovate or oblong, with an acute or cuneate and narrowed base, subentire-crenulate, crispy, glabrous, upto 30 (-45) cm. long. Peduncle upto 10-15 cm. long. Spathe lanceolate-oblong, purple on the outside, dark purple and blotched on the in side, upto 50 cm. long; tube ovoid; limb erect, lanceolate. Spadix as long as the spathe, with a 5-15 cm. long, terminal appendage. Fruit ovoid black.

Flowering and fruiting:	April-August
Distribution:	Gangetic Plains, Central India, Siwaliks, Punjab, Western Ghats and Himalayas (upto about 1650 m. alt.); generally in damp, shady, grassy localities, forest edges, ravine slopes and other place in the regions of occurrence.

Genus *Sauromatum* Schott. in family Araceae (about 115 genera with over 2,000 species in tropical and temperate regions, and abundant in tropics), with six species (in genus *Sauromatum* Schott.), distributed from tropical Africa to West Malesia (Malayasia), having herbs with a rhizome like corm. One species in Punjab, Gangetic Delta, Himalayas (upto 1650 m. alt. approximately) and Western Ghats in India where species growing in particular habitat.

Differential characters between two relevant genera of *Arisaema* Mart. and *Sauromatum* Schott. mainly based on the spadix with an apical and barren appendage in unisexual flowers; as *Arisaema* Mart. male flowers shortly pedicelled in plants usually dioecious, whereas the male flowers sessile in monoecious plants.

Sauromatum venosum (Aiton) Kunth. syn. ***Sauromatum guttatum*** Schott.Inflorescence short-stemned, foetid, with a large lanceolate conspicuously dark purple-blotched spathe, and a greenible yellow to dark purple, erect fleshy tapering spadix not quite as long. Spathe 32-50 cm., including the spathe-tube which is 8-10 cm., spathe-blade narrowed to a long slender, appearing in the autumn after flowering, pedate with 9-11 large unequal lanceolate leaflets; leafstalk mottled with black, up to 2 m. Corms large, flattened globular, c. 8 cm. across.

Flowering and fruiting: March-May

Distribution: Himachal Pradesh to Central Nepal, South-east Tibet, India; the regions between about 1000-2300 m. alt. in stony slopes and hot river valleys.

The genera in family Araceae are distinguishable on the basis of character of spadix with a flowerless apex-appendage or spadix covered with flowers to the apex-appendage absent; and the first of spadix is found in some genera such as *Arisaema, Sauromatum, Typhonium* and also others *(Thomsonia, Colocasia* which is also in other group having spadix covered with flowers to the apex and particularly leaves undivided). In the genus *Sauromatum,* the spathe with a short cylindrical tube and logy reflexed blade. spadix with very long appenadge male ad female flowers in widely separated zones and leaf one and pedate; and the *Suromatum* species (two) have male and female flowers on same spadix plant and base of spathe below whereas the spathe base not fused in other genera like ***Typhonium,*** and some others similar with these characters.

The tubers of the plant Sauromatum venosum (Ait.) Kunth. are medicinally useful; and the leaves are also utilised as vegetable.

Tubers are applied as stimulating poultice. Paste made with tuberous roots of the plant is applied over skin affections.For making external uses in tumours, the tubers or roots are pounded and made into a paste for applying over them. This is also topically applied to boils and other similar ailments.

Tubers are also edible and the leaves are made a vegetable preparation and eaten.

In addition, the tubers of this plant are considered useful in the veterinary medicine. Tubers are ground and pasted over the sores in animals and livestocks.

Bhasmakanda and Vajrakanda the Sanskrit names for the plant drug.

Vajrakanda (and synonyms allied to Vajraprokta), Susruta Samhita (Uttara. 60-48, variant) and Amaravarayudhahva (Susruta Samhita, Sutra. 46-305); Rakta-vajra-kanda and Vajraprokta (Dalhana, Susruta Samhita).

16

Tragia hispida Linn.

Tragia involucrata var. *cannabina* Muell.-Arg.

Family: Euphorbiaceae

Erect or climbing shrub, 4-5 ft. high, not twining, more or less hispid and with stnging hairs. Stems stout terete, woody, Leaves palmately 3-partite, upto 5.5 in. long, lobes toothed or pinnatifid the mid-lobe much longer than the lateral ones. Male flowers and calyx of female flowers similar to *T. involucrata.* Styles 3, slightly spreading, not revolute. Capsules 1/2 in. across, 3-lobed, hirsute, lobes globose. Seeds globose, smooth, 1/4 in. diam.

Throughout the hotter parts of India and in Ceylon. Bundelkhand, Yamuna ravines, nearby districts and other areas of region, in Uttar Pradesh, India.

Genus *Tragia* Linn. consisting species about 50, chiefly tropical species.

Tragia genus with salient characterstics- Styles united below in a stout column and continuous with the body of carpels; male calyx valvately 3-5-partite; stamens 3; fruit a capsule; twinning perenial herbs.

Flowering and fruiting: Rainy months, September-November

Major species of genus *Tragia* having relevance:

Tragia hispida Willd.

Tragia involucrata var. *angustifolia* Hook. f.

Tragia muelleriana var. **cordata** (Muell-Arg.) Pax & Hoffmann.

Tragia involucrata var. *cordata* Muell.-Arg.

Tragia plukenetii A.R. Smith.

Croton hastatus L.

C. unress L.

Tragia canabina L.f.

T. involucrata L. var. *canabina* Hook. f.

Tragia genus represented in the Peninsular India (Karnataka, Madras, Tamilnadu state and other areas in region). *Tragia hispida* Willd. in Western Peninsular India-Peninsular India-common in plains and hills in the eastern part; October-May. Former species with I leaves cordate at base with the former with 1 leaves acute at base. with hispid stinging hairs in both trailing or twining herbs, also straggling habit.

Micrococca mercurialis (Linn.) Benth.

Tragia mercutialis Linn.

Claoxylon mercurialis Thw.

Family: Euphorbiaceae

Regional names: Dondia (Hindi)

Annual herb upto 0.6 m. high. Leaves 3.6 x 2.3-3 cm., ovate, acute at apex, usually rounded at base, crenate. Racemes equalling or exceeding the leaves. Flowers short or long-pedicelled; the females flowers usually solitary and male flowers several. Capsules 4 mm. in diam., globose, glaborus or sparsely hairy, deeply 3-lobed, depressed. Seeds pitted.

Flowering and Fruiting:	Rainy season or June-August
	Plant found in Uttar Pradesh, the districts of Yamuna ravines in U.P., and other parts in central provinces, India.
Distribution:	Deccan Peninsula, Bihar and cultivation lands as weed. Burma, Ceylon, Arabia and Tropical Africa.

Tragia involucrata Linn.

Regional names: Barkanta (Hindi), Bichats (Bengla), Kamchhuri (Bombay state), Kammichi (Tamil), Dulagundi (Telgu), Choriyanum (Malayalam), Turachi (Kanarese), Dondia (Hindi)

Perennial more or less hispid herb, sub-scattered stinging hairs. Stems elongate, slender, twining. Leaves 1-4 in. long, variable, oblong, lanceolate to broadly ovate, acuminate, serrate, hairy, base rounded or cordate, petioles 1/2 in. or more long; stipules 1/2 in. long, ovate, acute, somewhat auricled at the base. Flowers yellowish, shortly stalked, usually in hairy racemes 1.2 in. long; bracts in long, lanceolate, acute. Male flowers sepals 3, pistillate minute, 3-fid. Female flowers sepals 6, ovate, pinnatifid, very hispid, elongating in fruit. Ovary 3-lobed, hispid; styles 3, united below in a stout column, often as long as the circinnately revolute branches. Capsule 1/2 in. diam, 3-lobed, white, hispid. Seeds gobose, smooth.

Throughout India from the Punjab and the outer Himalayan ranges eastwards to Assam; and southwards to Travancore and south to Burma, Southern India, Ceylon, China. Forests of North Oudh and Kheri districts in Uttar Pradesh, India.

Both species of *Tragia* may differ on main characterstics:

Tragia involucrata Linn. is a twining herb, with leaves single, and style circinately revolute; and *Tragia cannabina* Linn. ia as erect or sometimes climbing herb with leaves palmately 3-partite and styles slightly spreading not revolute.

Tragia hispida Willd. Petiole to 7 cm. long, blade 4-12x3.5 cm, ovate, acuminate, cordate, serrate. Perianth lobes hairy in female.

Tragia involucrata Linn. Petiole to 1 cm. long, blade 5-12x1-5 cm., linear-elliptic, entire or crenate-serrate.

The roots, leaves, fruits and whole plant of *Tragia involucrata* Linn. are medicinally useful.

Roots are diaphoretic and alterative, specially considered useful in the stage of fever when the extremeties are becoming cold; and also in pains in lower and upper limbs, or bodyache, in the form of infusion given in ardent fever and in itching of the skin. This infusion or decoction of roots of the plant is useful in different ailments and also as bitter tonic.

Fruits powder mixed with water considered for external use in baldness. The roots and whole plant in the form of powder, infusion and decoction useful in bronchitis, cramps, dysentery, cramps, dropsy, epilepsy, headache, madness, impotency or sexual debility, and also in cancer. Roots and fruits are useful in blood dysentery. Whole plant is useful in anasarca. Stems are useful in scabies, itching and similar skin-affections in internal use as infusion or powder; the roots are also useful, Leaves are useful in dysentery, rabid dog bite, swellings of limbs and other complaints as internal use. Roots are useful in snake bite.

The roots and other parts of *Targia canabina* Linn. and *Tragia mercurialis* Linn. are medicinally useful.

Tragia involucrata Linn. and *Tragia* species in relevance are considered among plant sources for Vṛscikālī, an important drug in indigenous medicine.

Vṛscikālī:	Caraka Saṁhitā, Vimān. 8-158; Cikitsā. 9-53, 10-32, 13-108, 16-119. Susruta Saṁhitā, Sutra. 38-4, 16, 38-7, 42-18. Aṣṭāṅga Hṛdaya, Sutra. 15-928; Cikitsa. 15-49, 16-37; Uttar. 2-10, 76, 6-36, 22-34 (and other allied drug and terms); and several works of Indian medicine.

17

Tricholepis glaberrima DC.

Family: Asteraceae (Compositae)

Regional names: Bismar, Brahmadandi, Ajadandi, Pirahdandi (Hindi), Motabor (Bombay),Ṽamanadandi (Bengla), Utateri Fusiyai (Gujarati)

Quite glabrous. Stem slender, erect, rigid, angled and ribbed. Leaves sessile, 2-3 in. long, linear-oblong or lanceolate, acute, entire or spinous-toothed, scaberulous and covered with raised points, prominently nerved, cauline leaves sometimes auricled at the base. Heads ovoid, 1/4-1/2 in. in diam. Involucre-bracts suberect, subulate, bristle pointed. Receptacle-bristles narrowly linear, exceeding the pappus. Achenes oblong, faintly ribbed, twice as long as the barbellate pappus.

Flowering and fruiting: Summers and onwards.

Distribution: Rajputana, Konkan, Deccan, Madhya Bharat, South Maharastra, Western Ghats, Bombay, South Kanara, Coorg and Mysore hills, Karnataks.

Plant occurring in Upper Gangetic plains, Uttar Pradesh, Madhya Pradesh, Rajasthan, Gujarat and other regions; usually on waste lands and fields or uncultivated farm lands and other various places in warm areas.

Tricholepis glaberrima DC. with specific characters mainly of stem elongate, slender and pappus and scabrid (not plumose), distinguished by *Tricholepis stictophyllum* Clark.

bearing short or O stem with plumose pappus or pappus hairs feathery alongwith other characters.

Tricholepis stictophyllum Clarke

Stictophyllum glabrum Edgew.

Cricus angustifolius Wall.

Subscapegerous glabrous perennial herb. Stem none or short, woods sparingly branched; branches angular, grooved, leafy below. Leaves amplexicaul, 3-5 in. long, linear or ligulate, acute, flat, entire or obscurely toothed, covered with minute raised pollute; nerves parallel to midrib. Heads solitary, or rarely 2 together at the naked end of branches glabrous, involucre bracts appressed glabrous outer ovate acuminate inner linear-lanceolate with erect flexous tips; corolla straight, pale-purple. Receptacle-bristles longer than the achenes. Achenes 1/3 in. long, pale, margins rounded, basal areole very oblique, linear-oblong, truncate, compressed, many-ribed, rather dilated at the apex, basal bracts quite oblique. Pappus plumose 1/3 in. long, silvery-brown, the hairs slightly united at the base.

Flowering and fruiting: March-April or spring-summers.

Western Himalaya, Sub Himalayan tracts, North Oudh Central India, Uttar Pradesh, Madhya Pradesh, Central Provinces, Upper Gangetic plains and adjoining areas in India; and in Upper Burma.

Tricholepis radicans (Roxb.) DC. Syn. *Cardus radicans* Roxb.

Erect annual herbs, upto 100 cm. Leaves at base obovate, and those above ovate to linear-lanceolate, crenate. Heads upto 0.7 cm. Florets purple.

Western Peninsular regions in India, common in western plains and upper Ghats (rocky grounds and usually on mountain slopes, Karnataka).

Flowering and fruiting: October-December

Amberoba ramosa (Roxb.) Jafri.

Cardus ramosus Roxb.

Volutrella divaricata (DC.) Benth.

Volutrella ramosa (Roxb.) Sant.

Oligochaeta ramosa (Roxb.) Wagenitz.

Microlonchus divaricatus DC.

Tricholenis procumbens Wight.

Centaurea divaricata Wall.

Family: Asteraceae (Compositae)

Regional names: Bhoyadandi (Hindi), Badaward (Persian), Sakayi (Marathi).

Straggling stiff annual dichotomously branched, glabrous or scaberulous; branches 1-2 ft. long. spreading, angled. Leaves very variable, sessile, 1-2 in-or longer, oblong or obevate. entire toothed or pinnatifid; lobes rounded and and mucronate, often undulate or crisped. Heads 1/3-1 in. long, 1/4-1/2 in. diam., glabrous or cottony pubescent. Involucre-bracts ovate or recurved with smooth spines the inner erect. Petals or receptacle short. Corolla 1/3 in. long, pale-purple; lobes linear, acute. Achenes acutely angled, grooved and punctate between the angles, base narrow, areole small, top broad and truncate achene 1/8 4-5 in. angled. Pappus of many unequal scaberulous silvery brown hairs, pappus spiny haris, innermost flattened and long.

Distribution: Central, Western and Southern India; from Bihar and the upper Gangetic plains to Lahore; and from Scind to Mysore and the Deccan, ascending to 3000 ft. in the north-west Himalayan region in India. Afghanistan and Baluchistan and other countries in the region.

Plant occurring commonly in various parts of Upper Gangetic plains on river banks, waste lands, ravinous and sandy soils areas in different parts of country.

Genus *Volutarella* Cass. in family Compositae, with species 4 or 5 in South Europe, North Africa, West Asia and India. Salient features of the genus-Annual. Leaves alternate. Heads heterogamous, purple-violet or blue. Outer flowers 1-seriate, neuter. Diskflowers 2-sexual, fertile; tube slender, short; limb cylindric, 5-fid. Involucre ovoid or globose; bracts many-seriate; innermost narrow, acute; outer shorter, acute-awned or spinescent. Receptacle flat, densely bristly. Filaments glabrous or hairy, bases sagitate; auricles connate, shortly tailed. Style filiform, arms free or connate. Achenes obvoid or oblong, subulate or angled, 5-15 ribbed, often striate and pitted between the ribs; basal areoles oblique or lateral. Pappus-bristles many-seriate outermost gradually shorter; innermost 2-4 dilated and flattened.

Genus *Volutarella* Cassine in tribe IX Cynaroideae (family Composittae) with main characters of all tubular flowers involucral-bracts many-seriate, spinous or foliaceous, imbricate, tips scarious; recepectacle densely bristly or paleaceous, rarely simply pitted; corolla-limb slender, deeply 5-fid; anthers-cells tailed; styles sub-entire, or arms short hairy or thickened towards the base; achenes often hard; pappus various, rarely O; leaves alternate, often spinous; common in several genera grouped in various subtribes; and the genus *Volutarella* in subtribe with heads 3 Centaureae separate, achenes glabrous, basal areole oblique or lateral, specifically with involucre not bracteate at the base or rarely so and characterstic of achenes terete, 10-15 ribbed in species which separate from relevant genera

Serratula Linn., *Tiricholepis* DC., *Centaurea* Linn. having main difference in filaments, anthers, and achenes in the species; whereas *Volutarella* Cass. characterised for heterogenous heads with fuseriate outer flowers, neuter and strongly 5-15 ribbed achenes.

Lamprachaenium microcephalum Benth.

Decaneuron microcephallum Dalz.

Family: Asteraceae (Compositae)

Regional names: Ajadandi, Biramdandi, Brahmadandi (Hindi), Bramhadandi (Bombay).

Erect branched annual, smelling, and with crisped hairs. Stem 1-2 ft., simple or branched from the base, glabrous hairy or glandular. Leaves petioled, 2-4 in., hairy above, white-tomentose beneath. Heads 1/4-1/3 in. diam.; peduncles slender; hispid of glabrate; involucral bracts acute, ciliate, none leafy, erect of recurved. Achenes 1/2 in.; pappus reddish, equalling the corolla-tube.

Distribution: Konkan, Southern Ghats, Bombay, Mabharastra, South Maharata and Mysore.

Dicoma tomentosa Cass.

Dicoma lanuginosa DC.

Acilepis lanata Spreng.

Discoma lanuginosa DC.

Xeropappus lanugginosus Wall.

Onopordon lanatum Herb.

Regional names: Biramdandi, Bhoydandi, Haranacana, Bajardanti, (Hindi-Gujarati),

Family: Asteraceae (Compositae)

Navanananjichapla, Choloharanacharo (Gujarat),

Annual, 10-18 in high, much branched, branches terete. Leaves 1-3 in., usually narrow, glabrate or cottonly above, nerves oobscrre. Heads glabrous; spines of involucre bracts yellowish, shining. Corolla 1/4 in. Achenes broad short, 1/8 in. long, turbinate, densely silky; pappus shining, elastics, inner membranous and hyaline with a rigid midrib, pale-brown 1/4 in. long, pappus longer than the achenes, outer bristle slender and inner longer, paleacuous.

Flowering and fruiting: Cold season; August-February. North-West India, Punjab Plains Western Peninsula, from the Konkan southwards, Tropical Africa; also Scind.

Plant occurring in Uttar Pradesh, Delhi, Rajasthan, Gujarat, Madhya Pradesh; Upper Gangetic Plains and adjoining regions: Jamuna and Chambal ravines, and central and northern India.

Dicoma tomentosa Cassini. Woody perennials up to 0.6 cm. Stem terete, white-hairy. Leaves alternate, 1-7 x 0.3-.5 cm., oblong, lanceolate, white-woolly beneath, hairy above. Heads solitary, homogamous. Florets white.

Tropical Africa, India; Western Peninsula; in plains on dry and gravelly terrains in Karnataka: Deccan, South Maharata, Carnatic, Nilgiris, Tamilnadu and other regions.

Genus *Dicoma* Cass. in family Compositae belonging to tribe IX Mutisiaceae (series I) with general features-Heads hetero or homogmous, rayed or not. Invol-bracts many-seriate (spinescent in *Dicoma* Cass.) Receptacle rarely paleaceous. Corolla deeply 5-fid, or 2-lipped. Anther-cells tailed. Style-arms rounded or truncate, not appendaged. Pappus various. Leaves usually alternate. Genus *Dicoma* Cass. with specific characters as Involucre-bracts spinescent particularly in this genus while other genera with many-seriate. Other main genera *Catamixis* Thoms. and *Leucomeris* Den. having tubular flower or 2-sexual or (in *Dicoma*) the outermost sometimes fem. and shortly ligulate; pappus-hairs simple in small tree of *Leucomeris* Den. and flowers all ligulate in small erect overgreen shrub of *Catamixis* Thoms.; whereas pappus-hairs feathery in small rigid shrub of *Dicoma* Cass.

Genus *Dicoma* Cass. Species 13 in Tropical and South Africa, one of which extends to India. Salient features of genus *Dicoma.* Cass Herbs, low shrub, annual or perennials, under shrub. Leaves alternate, entire. Heads solitary, subsessile on the branches, rarely corymbose, white or purple, homogamous, discoid, or heterogamous. Flowers all 2-sexual or heterogamous with the outer flowers female and all fertile, or the innermost sterile, tubular, limb, 5-partite, segments, erect or revolute; female (if present) slender with a short ligule. Involucral bracts many-seriate, ovate lanceolate, or linear, acuminate or spinescent, outer shorter, inner ones longer, broader, scarious along margin, all ending in long, scabrid spines; receptacle flat, naked glabrous, pitted. Outer fls. sometimes female. Anther-bases sagitate, fails long, bearded. Corolla tubular in both. 2-3 lobes in female. Style-arms obtuse. Achenes 10-ribbed, densely silky-villous, tipped by many feathery pappus hairs, outer pappus hairs some times scaly, shorter, paleaceous or of slender bristles.

The roots and whole herb of the plant *Tricholepis glaberrima* DC. are medicially useful.

Whole plant of *Tricholepis stictophyllum* Clarke. syn. *Cnicus angustifolium* Wall. *Trichelepis angustifolium* DC whole plant medicinally useful.

Whole herb of *Amberoba ramosa* (Rxb.) Jafri. syn. *Volutrella divaricata* (DC.) Benth. is medicinally useful.

Whole herb of *Lamprachaenium microcephalum* Benth. syn. *Deceaneuron microcephallum* Dalz. is medicinally useful.

Whole plant of *Dicoma tomentosa* Cass. syn. *Dicoma lanuginosa* DC. is medicinally useful.

Whole plant of *Tricholepis glaberrima* DC. is useful in leucoderma and skin diseases; considered nervine tonic and aphrodisiac, and useful in seminal debility.

Whole herb of *Amberoba divaricata* Kuntze. is useful as bitter tonic, aperient, deobstruent, febrifuge and blood purifier. Herb is slightly mucilaginous and useful in cough. Plant contains alkaloids.

Lamprachaenium microcephalum Benth. whole plant is useful as aromatic and bitter herb.

The roots of *Dicoma tomentosa* Cass. is applied topically in toothache and other tooth troubles.

Whole plant of *Amberoba ramosa* (Rxob.) Jafri. syn. *Oligochaeta ramosa* (Rxob.) Wagen. is useful in epilepsy and mental troubles.

The roots of *Tricholepis glaberrima* DC. are useful as antidote to snake-bite poison. Whole plant is useful in leprosy, menorrhagia and skin diseases.

Tricholepis graberrima DC. is source plant of Brahmadaṇḍī, an important drug in indiegnous medicine; and another or two plants *Amberoba ramosa* (Roxb.) Jafri. sy. *Volutrella divaricata* (DC.) Benth. is substitute source (Badavarda-Boyadandi in Unani medicine) Other two plants *Dicoma tomentosa* Cass. and *Lampraechaenicum microcephalum* Benth. are among the adulterants, substitues or relevant botanical sources for Brahmadaṇḍī and allied plant drugs.

Medicinal properties and actions of the plant drug-Tikta katu rasa, Katu vipāka, Uṣṇa vīrya; Kaphavāta sāmaka; Sothahara, Vedanāsthāpana, Raktasuddhikara, Tvacya, Svedajanana, Dāhaprasamana, Ropaṇa, Sajñāsthāpana, Kaṭupauṣṭika, Smṛtijanan, Kāsahara, Stambhana, Javarahara, Soṇitaprasādana, Nāḍībalya; and therpeutically indicated in fever, periodic or remmittent fever, Oedema, skin affections, epilepsy, insanity (Jvara, niyatakālika Jvara, sotha, tvacavikāra, apasmāra, unmāda), madhumeha (diabetes), prameha (urinary disorders), Nāḍīdaurbalya (nervine debility), Cittabhramsa (giddiness and mental trouble), Atyārtavá (menorrhagia), Atisāra (diarrhoea) Yakrdvikāra (liver disorders). Kasa (cough), Sukrameha (spermatorrhoea), and Vātaroga and Vṛṇa (ulcers or wounds) specially in chronic ulcer or wounds delaying in healing; and also in swelling, particularly seeds are applied over inflammed parts of body.

Whole herb of the plant drug is burnt to ash and finely prepared an ointment by mixing in oil or similar base which is externally and regularly applied over chronic ulcers or wounds where the healing is delayed. Seeds are powdered and pasted over swelling.

Leaves of drug are expressed for obtaining the juice which is mixed with honey. This paste is useful for applying in vagina (yoni lepa) for enhancing the sexual satisfaction in coitus (viṣayānanda) as recipe prescribed (Vaidyamanoramā, Guhya roga cikitsadhikara).

The powder or infusion of whole plant of drug is given in cases of Madhumeha or diabetes regularly as an effective remedy.

Similarly the infusion or decoction, juice and powder also usually used in skin diseases as blood purifier, mental complaints, spermatorrhoea, cough and other various complaints under therapeusis.

Brahmadaṇḍī: Rājanighaṇṭu, Parpaṭādī varga, 133; Nighaṇṭuratnākara

18

Tridax procumbens Linn.

Family: Asteraceae (Compositeae)

Local names: Ghamra, Baramasi (Hindi)

Annual or prennial herb, weak straggling, pubescent or hispid of 1-3 ft. height. Leaves few, petioled, 1-2 in. long, ovate or lanceolate, coarsely cordate or pinnatiscent, clothed on both sides with bulbous based haris. Peduncles often more than one found long, solitary, sparsely pilose. Heads 1/4 in. diam; outer invol-bracts densely hairy, ovate, acuminate; inner longer, membranous, slightly pubescent on the back. Ligules of ray-flowers yellow, 3-partite; anthers brown. Pappus of many shining feathery bristles.

Common plant throughout India. Abundant in the Gangetic plains in northern India (by roadsides, in grassy places and old walls and other places in the provinces). Indigenous to central America.

Tridax procumbens Linn. An erect or straggling, hispid herb. Leaves or lanceolate, dentate or pinnatisect. Heads creamy or shitish, long peduncled, about 1 x 1.5 cm. Achenes brown. Plant abundantly found all over in waste places, along roadsides and in the cervices of old walls in the plains in north India; Punjab, Delhi, Haryana and other many areas in country. Pantropical plant as common weed in open places, Karnataka, Tamilnadu, Southern India.

Tridax procumbens L. Procumberrt herbs, creeping and ascending. Petiole short, hairy; leaf blade 2.5-4 x 1.5 — 7.5 cm., acute, deeply incise-dentate, sometimes 3-lobed, lobes acute, hairs thick-based. Heads to 1.2 cm., outer bracts ovate, acute, herbaceous, green, pubescent, inner bracts scarious, pinkish above middle. Corolla yellow. Growing as common weed in Karnataka and Madras.

Flowering and fruiting: Greater part of the year or all seasons; December-May or various months.

Genus *Tridax* Linn. Species 7, native of south America out of which one has become naturalised in India. Distinguishing characters of genus in family: Flowers white, spinescent; heads peduncled; Pappus scales awned and plumose, ligules of ray florets large; pappus of short of long aristate, feathery bristles or bristle plumose.

Tridax Linn. genus belonging to group II Tubuliflorae and tribe 8 Mutisieae with ray and usually disc florets bilabiate and *Tridax* Linn. falls under genera having flowers white, whitish or creamy in colour; heads simple, leaves simple, involueral bracts not spinescent, heads short or long peduncled, and specially pappus scales awned and plumose; ligules of ray florets large, marginal flowers 5-6, with pale-yellow or white and corolla of disc flowers bright yellow, whereas the flowers with pale yellow, orange-yellow, greenish yellow, pale or bright blue and other colour and shades found in several other genera; and mainly flower colour in *Tridax* Linn. usually yellow (corolla) with varying colour in other parts of flower, in the plants varying colour in other parts of flower, in the plants occurring in different regions of country.

Tridax procumbesn Linn. Procumbent- ascending, annual-biennial, somewhat patently hispid herbs. Stems branched, creeping at base, suberect or trailing above. Leaves on 0.5-2 cm. long petioles, ovate-lanceolate, or elliptic-rhomboid, with a cuneate base, obtuse or subacute, coarsely serrate or lobed, patently hispid, 2.5-7 x 0.6-4 cm. Heads solietary, on erect, patently long-pilose, 10-30 cm. long peduncles, 1.2-1.5 cm., across. Involucral bracts 2 to 3-seriate, outer ones ovate-lanceolate, acuminate, hairy; inner ones lanceolate, 0.6-0.7

cm. long, thinly hairy. Marginal flowers 5-6, with pale-yellow or white, 3-dentate, 0.3 cm. long ligules. Corolla of disk-flowers bright yellow, 0.5 cm, long with hariy, recurved segments. Achenes pilose, 0.2 cm. long. Pappus-bristles 15-20, unequal, 0.50.7 cm. long. Palea 0.8-1 cm. long.

Commonly growing in different kinds of habitats in various parts of country such as river-beds, readsides, waste places, grassy localities, fields or farms, forest edges, forest clearings, gardens and other many places, as one of the common weeds in areas of species occurrence.

The main parts of the plants-having medicinal utility are leaves and whole plant. Chiefly this plant has been easily available for fresh wounds and ulcers including cuts, bruises and other similar injuries resulting deep cuts over skin of body parts and bleeding from incised wounds of different kinds and stages. Whole plant, specially leaves including tender branches or stems, if necessary for supplemening the quantity of leafy raw material, are taken afresh preferably and washed with clean water for making the herb free from soils and any other dirty substance (as sterlised or disinfectant herbal receipe is desirable for applying over the wounds and ulcers which are normally required to be prevented from any kind of infection or septic). This herbal material is ground or pounded on stony slate or any other apparatus or equipment (like grinder) and the paste prepared finely is applied topically over wounds, ulcers, cuts or affected part with lesion, and proper bandage and dressing are provided in case the same is required depending upon the degree and condition or ailment under treatment by the herbal medicament. In condition of non-bandaged wounds, the paste with thick coat over the injured region is made and permitted to dry up for little or adequate time, with or without bandage and application of cotton or gauze (otherwise completely clean cloth pieces). Normally small or ordinary wounds, ulcers or cuts are simply treated with herbal paste, and rest all other major or bigger injuries and ulcers are given full dressing with extra care. Further change of drug application is made with usual dressing in forthcoming period of illness, and this process continues till the ulcer or injured part heals up speedily and completely with a few days or minimum time of healing of such wound or ulcer.

This is quite effective herbal cure against the ulcers, wounds and injuries caused with sharp instruments, weapons or implements, and also wounds and ulcers including boils and abscess (and other various ailments of this group) as a highly responsive medicament of the plant possessing healing, styptic, antiseptic and anodyne and other properties in medicinal efficacy relevant for treatment of ulcers and wounds as this herbal application is potent to check bleeding and stopping haemorrhage and to help faster healing of injury and also healing even those of incised wounds there could not be properly stitched up for lack of facilities or due to emergency; as sometimes no remarkable scar remains in ordinary lesions.

On account of various medicinal properties such as haemostatic or styptic, antiseptic, wound healer, astringent and allied potentialities, the plant, leaves, stems, branches and other parts like roots and lowers are useful in the plant treatments of ulcers, wounds, blisters, boils, cuts, sores and other ailments of this category which may be therapeutically managed through the application of this plant in various forms and recipes applied generally in external administration of single drug formula basically which can be found in use as for added or modified with other ingridients for suitability and enhancing usability and effectiveness.

In skin diseases, eczema, leprosy and other similar type of dermatological affections on body skin, the roots and leaves are useful as external application in the form of expressed juice, paste or by rubing like ointment or cream over the affected part with skin complaints or dermatological problems; and also decoction of various parts or whole plant may be applicable for external wash or application on skin ailments of various kinds.

The leaves are also useful to apply over painful teeth in form of leaves-paste or leaves expressed juice is dropped in condition of toothache; and the leaves-juice is also helpful to cure mouth sores or stomatitis and sometimes with gum-boil or similar complaints. Among other external usses of the plant, the application of leaves, stems and whole plant in the form of juice, infusion after poisonous stings or bite like scorpion-stings and bee-stings (and also other insects).

Expressed juice of leaves or whole plants in quantity of 3-5 teaspoonful or half cup of tea, mixed with water or any other medicinal decoction is internally useful in some diseases such as urinary calculus or stone in urinary bladder and stomach disorders, fever, diarrhoea, dysentery and other similar complaints of digestive system or alimentary canal. In case of fever and stomach troubles particularly stomachache, the slight warm water may be suitable vehicle, mixed with Juice, about 5-10 ml. In comparison the infusion is preferable for preparation of medicinal receipe from fresh herbal material, and the decoction or powder may be prepared from dried raw material though the green herb is frequently found due to its easy and wide approachability for plant source. Other than human ailments, the plant is also useful in veterinary medicine. Paste of whole plant or leaves and stems is externally applied over sores, ulcers or wounds in amimals and cattles. Similarly the plant paste application over the injured part of animal body with any kind of incised wound may be useful in treatment of wounds, ulcers and cut-injuries in livestocks and animals.

Plant drug is easily procurable from field where the source herb is abundantly grown as a common weed during rainy season and other months practically throughout the year in the areas where plant thrives on every type of soils specially in grass lands, roadsides, river banks, crop field and old walls and many other localities. Collection of plant for medicinal use may be made at any time or at the time of fair growth is usually after the rains. Preferably the collection of plant material for effective medicinal potentiality, the raw drug is procurable after flowering and fruiting are over as common pattern, for maximum potency.

Pīta Bhṛṅgarāja, the kind of Bhṛṅgarāja, a major drug of indigenous system of medicine. *Eclipta alba* Hassk. and *Wedelia calendulacea* Less. (both plants in Asteraceae) are botanical sources for Bhṛṅgarāja and Pīta bhṛṅgarāja respectively; and the plant *Tridax procubens* Linn. another kind or source of Pīta bhṛṅgarāja, also as substitute medicinal plant for specific therapeutic indications.

Three kinds or varieties (jāti or bheda) or Bhṛṅgarāja Sveta (white), Pīta (yellow) and Nīla-Kṛṣṇa (blue-black) in Rāja Nighaṇṭu (satāhvādi varga, 138-140).

Bhṛṅgarāja (Bhṛṅga and Mārkava): Caraka Samhita (Cikitsa. 4-67, 18-116, 26-262, Kalpa. 1-28), Susruta Samhita (Cikitsa. 25-28, Kalpa. 8-54, 56; Uttar. 39-224, 51-29), Astanga Hardaya (Uttar. 24-37, 42; 39-162). Rāja Nighaṇṭu (ṣatāhvādi varga, 136-140), Bhāvaprakāsa Nighaṇṭu (Guḍūcyādi varga, 239), Kaiyadeva Nighaṇṭu (oṣadhi varga, 1573-1575) and several works of indigenous medicine.

19

Typhonium trilobatum Schott.

Typhonium triste Griff.

Arum trilobatum Linn.

Typhonium siamense Engler.

Arisaema pumiilum Blume.; *A. pumilum* Lamk.

T. orixens Schott.

Family: Araceae

Regional name: Gada (Hindi), Cheikochu (Bengla), Chena (Malayalam), Karunaikhihangue (Tamil), Kandagadde (Telgu), Ghet-kachhu.

Tuber subglobose. Leaves 5-12. diam; lobes ovate; petiole 1 ft. or shorter. Peduncle 1-4 in. Spathe 8-12 in.; limb upto 1/2 in., broad, red purple inside, nearly flat, tip not twisted. Appendage bright red, stout or slender.

Distribution: Lower Bengal, Burma, the Eastern and Western Peninsula and Ceylon. Siam, Malay Islands.

Genus *Typhonium* Schott.-Species about 13, tropics of the Old World. Limb of spathe broadly ovate, open, narrowed into a long point.

Typhonium trilobatum Schott.

An erect, stemless tuberous herb; tubers creamy white to pale brown. Leaves radical, hastately 3-lobed or tripartite, long-petioled 20-27 cm. long, reticulately veined, entire. Spathes ovate, narrowned into along point, purplish; Flowers bisexual.

Plant found in Madhya Pradesh, India.

Distribution: Genus *Typhonium* in Tropics of the World, Konkan, South Konkan and Western Peninsula, Chhota Nagpur, Central Bengal, Eastern Bengal, Chittagong, Eastern coast of the Madras state and Singhbhumi.

Typhonium genus and species mistakenly may resemble with genus *Amorphophallus* which may be broadly differentiated by its tubers depressed-lobose, 25-30 cm., across, leaves twice bifold while tubers sub-globose, smaller, leaves hastately tripartite in genus *Typhonium* and species.'

Genus *Typhonium.* Spath with a short tube and long blade which is deciduous; spadix with elongate smooth appendage; male and female flowers in separate zones. Leaves variable. Two species, is *Typhonium trilobatum* (L.) Schott. and another *Typhonium diversifolium* Walkich ex Schott. in family Araceae (a large family of pan-tropical herbaceous plants with a few temperate species).

Typhonium diversifolium Wallich ex Schott.

Family: Araceae

Herb with aerial stems with underground tubers. Leaves are quite variable as its name implies, leaves being either entire, heart-shaped, arrow-shaped, spear-shaped, or with 5-7 lanceolate to linear lobes. Spathe green outside, variously striped, spotted or netted with dark reddish-purple within, variable in size 5-20 cm., with a short green tube and lanceolate finely-pointed blade. Spadix ending in a blunt cylindrical dark purple appendage to c. 8 cm. long, which protrudes from, oris enclosed in the longer spathe. Leaves usually solitary, appearing with the inflorescence, 8-13 cm. broad and long. Corm upto 2 cm. in diameter.

Flowering and fruiting: July-August

Distribution: Himachal Pradesh to South-east Tibet; the Himalayan ranges from 2500-4300 m. alt., in shrubberies and open slopes.

The plants belonging to Araceae or Arum family, with aerial stems or with underground tubers or rhizomes, and with a very distinctive unique, often foetid inflorescence which attracts flies and other insects; inflorescence comprising a large spathe often conspicious coloured, subtending, or encircling and often fused below round a fleshy central axis, bearing numerous tiny inconspicuous flowers, either covering the spadix, or borne only round the basal part; the sterile apical part of the spadix, the appendage, often well-developed; flowers bisexual or unisexual. Various genera and their species show the difference and similarity in regard to salient features of these member species.

Two major division of family on the basis of main characters of spadix may be done, and a group of plants bearing spadix wuth a flowerless apex-the appendage relating male and female flowers presence. In *Arisaema* genus the male and female are flowers on different plants but these are on same plant spadix in the genera *Typhonium, Sauromatum* and some other genera. Further these two relevent genera differ for base of spathe which is fused below into a tube in genus *Sauromatum* when the same is not fused in genus *Typhonium.*

The roots or bulbs of plant *Typhonium trilobatum* Schott. are medicinally useful and edible as vegetable.

Bulbs contain sitosterol, two unidentified sterols and a crystalline compound.

Roots are stimulant and used for piles. Bulbous roots are eaten with bananas in stomach complaints.

The tubers of the plant are considered useful in snake-bite cases, and both external as well as internal uses are made in this condition. For oral application, the tubers are cut into the slices and 2-3 slices or small pieces are to be given initially which fluctuate in quanity keeping in view of severity, stage and symptoms in snake bitten person and venomous effect and its extent. In lieu of tubers slice, the expressed juice about 2-3 teaspoonful may also be given alone or with slice at an interval of half to one hour in low or increased quantity and frequency of in-take; and gradually the oral use of tuber may be reduced in quanity frequency and interval in process of tuber internal administration. Simaltaneously the tubers are pounded and paste is made; and it is externally applied over snake bitten part of body (lesion). The usual measures required in snake bite cases are followed in regard to bandage, ligature and all other essential process.

Tuberous roots of the plant may be collected during rains or autumn, and kept after drying in shade, for medicinal uses. Fresh tubers are procured from the areas of occurrence and slices particularly juice may be readily obtained and internally used medicinally.

Agadakanda, the Sanskrit name for *Typhonium trilobatum* (L.) Schott.

20

Ventilago denticulata Willd.

Ventilago calyculata Tulsane.

Ventilago madraspatana Gaertn. var. *calyculata* (Tul.) King.

Family: Rhamnaceae

Regional names: Bongasarjom, Raidhui, Ghurbela, Kevli, Kanyel (Bombay), Raidhani (Hindi), Kuriyadai (Kanada) Pinchuli, Kalibel; Kuktupita (Bengla),

Large climbing shrub with wooly tendrils, young parts and inflorescence pubescent. Leaves 2-4 in., petioled, elliptic-oblong from an oblique base, acute or acuminate, entire or crenate, glabrous when mature; main lateral nerves 6-8 pairs, aronate. Flowers many, small, greenish, with an offensive smell, in long terminal leafless panicles; petals deflexed. Nut subglobose, 1/4 in. diam., girt about the middle by the rim of the calyx-tube, wing linear, pubescent, terminated by the remains of the bifid style.

Flowering and fruiting: February-March; April-June (fruits ripening May-June).

Distribution: Sub-Himalayan tracts from the Jamuna to Nepal; also in Bengal, Central India, Western Ghats, Bhutan and Burma extending to Java.

Ventilago madraspatana Gaertner. Scandent shrubs. Leaf-blade upto 5.2 x 2 cm., oblong-elliptic, shortly acute. Flowering and fruiting stages during the period from

December to April or till summers. Western Peninsular India, Sri Lanka, Java. Common in plains and Ghats, in deciduous and semi-evergreen forests, Karnataka, India.

Ventilago madraspatana Gaertn. Syn. *Ventilago bracteata* Wall. Young branches and leaves glabrous or only slightly pubescent. Leaves 2-4 by 1-1.5 in., oblong-lanceolate to ovate, acute, or subacuminate, crenate or entire; costal narves 6-8 pairs. Calyx slightly puberulous outside, glabrous inside; ovary with a few white hairs at the base; styles nearly straight. Flowers in simple or paniculate spikes; fruits nut girt at the base.

Regional names: Pitti (Raktavalli (Hindi), Raktapita (Bengla), Ellasurugndu Lekhandi (Bombay), Pappali (Kanarese), Pappīli (Tamil).

Western Peninsula, from the Konkan Southwards, Tennasserin, Ceylon; common in dry places. Maharastra, Tamilnadu, Deccan and Karnataka in India.

Ventilago calyculata Tulasne. Syns. *Ventilago denticulata* Willd *Ventilago macrantha* Tulasne., *Ventilago madraspatana* Roxb. Leaves pubescent, ovate or ovate-elliptic, crenate-serrate, with about 5 pairs of costal nerves. Calyx densely pubescent without, hairy within on the disk. Flowers in densely pubescent paniculate spikes; ovary densely pubescent, styles longer and more divulging. Fruit yellow, often densely pubescent, at length, nut girt round the middle. Variable plant in size of leaves and amount of pubescence.

Throughout the hotter parts of India, from the Kumaon and Nepal to Bhutan, Sylhet, Tenasserim, and throughout the Western Peninsula; Java.

Genus *Ventilago* Gaertner. Unarmed, climbing shrubs. Leaves crenate-serrate, pinnately veined, oblique at base. Flowers small, disposed in axillary and terminal (usually leafless panicles, namely the axils of lvs. Calyx lobes keeled within; petals emarginate. Anther connectives produced. Disc flat, sunk in calyx tube, angled. Ovary half-inferior, 2-locular; styles, flat. Fruit 1-locular, nutlike, with linear-oblong wing. Seeds subglobose exalbuminous. Species about 10 scattered over the tropics of Asia, Africa, America, Australia, and the Pacific Islands.

Genus *Ventilago* Gaertner in family Rhamnaceae (species over 400 inhabiting tropical and temperate parts of the world) with fruit indehiscent, peduncled above into a linear-oblong wing whereas another genus *Smythes* Seeman. (both genera in tribe Ventilagineae) fruit a 2-valved broadly oblong capsule.

Specific characters of Genus *Ventilago* Gaertner of plants unarmed with styles 2, persisting to form a wing on fruit, differs from *Sageretia* Brongniart for styles 3, decidous and its fruit without winges.

Broadly the genus *Ventilago* Gaertn. with salient features a woody climber with dry fruit, indehiscent, winged, 1-celled, ovary 1/2 inferior or nearly superior; comparatively in distinction with other related genera.

The bark, young shoots, root bark, fruits, seeds, and whole plant of *Ventilago denticulata* Willd. syn. *Ventilago calyculata* Tul. are medicinally useful.

In malarial fever, the juice of bark and young shoots of the plant are applied over body for bodyache or generalised pain in body parts. Other parts are also medicinally used in different complaints. *Ventilago calyculata* Tulsane is therapeutically useful in various forms.

The powder of roots bark of *Ventilago madraspatana* Gaertn. is useful as carminative, stomachic, stimulant and given in atonic dyspepsia, debility and in mild fevers. Bark powder is mixed with gingelly oil used as an application in skin affections, itches and similar skin complaints.

Root bark of *Ventilago madraspatana* Gaertn. contains trihydroxymethyl-anthrasnolmonomethyl ether, and emodinmonomethyl ether.

The various parts of the plant *Ventilago denticulata* Willd. are useful in different ailments. Whole plant is useful in syphilis, veneral diseases and urinary disorders, dysuria, Wood sap is useful in ear complaints in pus condition and earache. Roots are considered antidote to snake-bite poison. Bark powder is useful as cooling medicine. Stems and whole plant are useful in eye complaints and night blindness (in proper form of application). Whole plant is useful in skin affections and scabies, and also in fever. Stems and roots are useful in headache. Bark is useful in rheumatism, peptic ulcer, stomach complaints and spermatorrhoea. Bark is also applied to sprains. Whole plant is useful in urinary complaints specially retention of urine. Seeds oil is edible. Seeds are considered abortifacient.

Internal and external modes or administration in various forms of decoction, infusions, powder, paste, lotion, juice and other kinds of usage.

Parts used (upādeyāṅga) roots (mūla), bark (tvak), fruit (phala), whole plant (pañcāṅga), stem (kāṇḍa), seeds (bīja) and others (anya aṅga).

Tāmravallī, Lohitayastika, Ramataruni (ramataruni), and Kaivartikā, the Sanskrit names for *Ventilago madraspatana* Gaertn.

Kaivarttikā: Raja Nighantu, Guducyadi varga, 119 Tamravalli: Susruta Samhita. Sutra. 10-59: Aṣṭāṅga Hṛdaya, Sārīr. 2-54, Uttar. 35-46.

Lohitayastikā: Lohita: Susruta. Cikitsā. 11-9.

Aṣṭāṅga Hṛdaya, Cikitsā. 19-38, 21-68; Kalpa. 4-12; Uttar. 5-9, 27-38.

Section - II

1

Acalypha indica Linn.

A. *spicata* Forsk.

A. *ciliata* wall.

A. *canescense* wall.

Regional names: Kuppu (Hindi), Kuppigida (Kannarese), Muktajhuri (Bengla), Vanchi kanto (Bengla) Kunkimphal (Konkan), Khokli (Marathi), Kuppiveni (Tamil), Kuppichettu (Telgu), Kuppumani (Malayalam), Dodano (Gujarati), Indian Acalypha (English); Kuppameni, Khokali.

Erect annual herb, 1-2.5 ft. high. Branches many, angular, finely pubescent. Leaves thin, glabrous, 1-3 in. long, ovate or rhomboid-ovate, obtuse or subacute, crenate-serrate; base cuneate, 3-nerved; petioles slender, usually longer than the blade; stipules minute. Flowers in lax erect axillary elongate spikes; the makes minute, clustered towards the summit of spike, ebracteate; the females in clustered of 3-5 subtended by a shortly stalked leaf-like truncate dentate many-nerved bract. Capsules hispid concealed by the bracts, often only 1-seeded. Seed 1/10 in. long, ovoid, smooth, pale-brown.

Flowering and fruiting: Flowering during greater part of the year; September-June

Distribution: Throughout the hotter parts of India and in Ceylon, extending to Java and Tropical Africa Very common in the areas of Upper Gangetic Plains, especially as a garden weed.

Acalypha indica Linn.

Erect herbaceous annual, 30-80 cm. high, with many spreading or ascending branches. Leaves membranous, 5 x 3.5 cm., ovate or rhomboid-ovate, crenate-serrate, cuneate at base, arranged in a mosaic. Flowers minute, green, in lax, erect, axillary spikes; males clustered towards the top; females fls. solitary or paired, each enclosed by foliar, 5x5 mm. bract. Capsules concealed by persistent bracts. Seeds ovoid, pale brown, shining.

Plant occurring as common plant as a garden weed in the shades of tress and shrubs; and also found in waste places and in cultivated fields; Delhi area, Haryana, Punjab and adjoining areas; northern India.

Acalypha indica Linn. Annual 1-3 ft. Leaves 1-2 in., acute or obtuse, base cuneate entire; petals slender, often longer than the blade. Spikes 1-3 in., slender, erect bracts 1/4-1/2 in. diam., cuneiform, many-nerved. Ovary hispid. Capsules spike concealed by the bract, often only 1-seeded, hispid. Seed ovoid, acute, smooth.

Hotter parts of India from Bihar eastewards to Assam and southwards to Singapore and Burma; and from the Ceylon to Travancore. Ceylon, common in fields. Westwards to Tropical Africa, and eastwards to Timor and the Phillippines.

Acalypha ciliata Forsk.

A. fimbriata Schum.

A. ciliata Herb.

A. nubra Herb.

Family: Euphorbiaceae

Annual 1-2 ft., rather stout, glabrous or pubescent. Leaves 2-3 in., sometimes caudate acuminate, base cuneate or rounded; petiole usually longer than the blade. Spikes rarely 1 in. long; bracts (like the calyx of a Labiatae plant), hispid or glabrous, pale, teeth as long as the limb. Ovary spinely hispid. Capsule glabrous; cocci very thin, white, glabrous, twisted after dehiscence. Seeds globosely ovoid, nearly smooth.

Flowering and fruiting: August-November

Distribution: Western Himalaya, 3000-6000 ft. elevation, from Kashmir to Garhwal. The Deccan Peninsula, Ceylon, Arabia, Tropical Africa.

Acalypha ciliata Forsk.

Erect, often much-branched, annual herbs. Stems ribbed, hairy. Leaves ovate-rhomboid, with a rounded-subcordate or cuneate base, crenate-serrate, 5-10 x 2-6 cm. Petioles 3-8 (-10) cm. long Inflorescence finally elongates up to 2 cm. long, with 4-8 (-12), male bracts at base and a cluster-like or spiciform male upper part. Females bracts 0.2 cm. long, patent-hairy, ribbed, dentate with 20 ciliate teeth, accrescent in fruiting. Perianth-segments 3, ovate, acute. Fruits enclosed by the accrescent bract. Seeds smooth, male flower stamens 8.

Plant commonly occurring along waysides, roadsides and in agricultural fields; Siwaliks, Dehradun and adjacent areas; Upper Gangetic Plains, Bundelkhand, Uttar Pradesh, Madhya Pradesh and other various areas in the region. Maharastra, Bengal.

Acalypha malabarica Mueller

A. hispida Heyne.

Family: Euphorbiaceae

Regional names: Vattattali (Malayalam)

Annual hairy herbs. Blade 1-3 x 1-1.5 cm., ovate, crenate-serrate, palmately 5-ribbed. Spikes axillary, female fls. 2-3 in the axils of large, folded, toothed, pink bracts; teeth with gland-tipped hairs. Ovary pilose, hairy.

Flowering and fruiting: September-November

Distribution: Central and Peninsular India. Fairly common in plains, in open country or around cultivated fields, Karnataka; Tamilnadu, Southern India.

Acalypha malabarica Muell.-Arg.

A rather stout leafy annual 4-6 in., stem stout. Leaves 1.5-2 in, base cuneate, glabrous; petiole longer than the blade. Spikes 1.5 in., male portion with few minute glabrous flowers. Bracts 1/8 in., broad, separated by short intervals. Seeds globosely ovoid, obscurely granulate.

Acalypha malabarica Muell.-Arg. Herbaceous, flaccid, stem pubescent, leaves long-petioled, ovate subacute subterrate, spikes all axillary sessile short androgynous, male fls. very few, terminal minute 3-7 altlernate, 2-5 fid, glabrous, many-toothed and bordered with slender gland-tipped hairs rather longer than the capsules.

Acalypha fruticosa Forsk.

A. capitata Wall.

A. amentaceae Roxb.

A. betulina Retx.

Family: Euphorbiaceae

Regional names: Sinni, Sinni-morum (Tamil), Chinni (Deccan, Telgu), The Birch-Leaved Acalypha (English)

Bushy plant 4-8 ft. high, strong-smelling shrub, more or less covered with yellow waxy glands; shoots and spikes pubescent. Leaves 1-3 in., crenate, obtuse or subacute, base usually acute; petiole much shorter than the limb. Spikes 1/4-1 In., solitary, bracteate and 2-lanceolate, usually male with a few female flowers at the base. Sepals of male pubescent. Ovary hairy and glandular, styles with filiform arms. Capsules tomentose. Seeds smooth.

Distribution:	Deccan Peninsula. Pegu, Martaban, Ava, Ceylon, Arabia and Tropical Africa.
Flowering and fruiting:	Beginning of the hot season and onwards.

Acalypha alnifolia Kleis.

A. capitata Willd. & Muell.

Family: Euphorbiaceae

Small shrub. Leaves 1-2 in., sometimes orbicular almost, base rounded or subcordate variable in hairiness; petiole rarely half the length of the blade. Male spikes 1-3 in.; female spikes of few obtusely lobed imbricating bracts. Sepals of male fls. pubescent. Capsules hispid. Seeds subglobose.

Distribution:	Deccan Peninsula

Acalypha alnifolia Klein.

Shrubby plant; stem pubescent and often ciliate with long deciduous hairs; leaves ovate acute serete pubescent above and usually tomentose beneath; male spikes axillary slender dense-fid, females terminal sessile capitate; bracts 1-fid, 6-9-toothed capillary branches.

Acalypha brachystachya Hornem.

A. conferta Roxb.

A. calyciformis Wall.

A. fissa Herb.

Family: Euphorbiaceae

Herbaceous, flaccid, nearly glabrous annual, 6-12 in. Leaves long-petioled ovate orovate-cordate, subacute, crenate-serrate, spikes all axillary sessile very short, androgynous, male fl. very few terminal minute, females bracts few 2-3-fid, crowded at the base of the spike very large cut into 3 linear 1-nerved obtuse lobes, styles pectinately laminate.

Leaves 1-3 in., membranous, acute obtuse or acuminate; petiole often longer than the blade. Bracts forming axillary clusters each 1/4-1/2 in. long; lateral segments shorter, all spreading Male flowers in minute clusters on the very short filiform apex of the spike. Capsules hispid, quite concealed in the large green bracts. Seeds subglobose nearly smooth.

Flowering and fruiting:	September-November
Distribution:	Java and Tropical Africa. Temperate Himalaya, 4,000-8,000 ft. elevation; from Kashmir to Nepal; Khasia hills, 4,000 ft. alt. Deccan Peninsula, from Canara southwards; Ceylon.

Acalypha brachystachya Hornem.

Erect, often much-branched, somewhat flaccid, annual herbs. Stems sulcate, thinly patently hairy. Leaves ovate, with a subcordate base, acute-acuminate, crenate, thinly hairy, 2-4 (-6) x 1-3 (-4) cm. Petioles 2.5-5 (-6) cm. long. Inflorescence short, axillary, 1-2 cm. long, finally, with 2-6 (-10). Male fls. bracts at base, and a short, cluster-like or spiciform. Female fls. upper part. Male flowers bracts 1 to 2 flowered; 0.4-0.6 (-0.7) cm. long; segments oblong lanceolate, oblong, gland-ciliate, 1-nerved. Perianth-segments ovate, acute, ciliate. Fruit depressed-globose, hairy, ± 2 cm. across. Seeds smooth. Female fls. calyx-segments 4, ovate, acute. Stamens 8.

Plant found in the Upper Gangetic Plains; Dehradun, herbs along the way sides or waste places in open or shady situation in the area and humid localities of ravines

Acalypha racemosa Wall. ex Benth.

A. *paniculate* Miq.

A. *filiformis* Heyne.

A. *wallichiana* Thwaies.

A. *racemosa* Heyne.

Family: Euphorbiaceae

Undershrub or herb, finely pubescent. Leaves 2-6 in., coarsely unequally crenate-serrate; petiole 1-4 in. Male spikes solitary, 2-6 in., dense-fid, female racemes or apneicles capillary; bracts-scattered, 3-fid, ovate, obtuse, shorter than the pedicels. Sepals of female gland-ciliate, ovate-lanceolate, at length reflexed. Capsules 1/10 in. diam., 3-lobed, glandular; styles 3-7 partite. Seeds reticulately pitted.

Distribution: Deccan Peninsula; from Malabar southward; Ceylon, ascending to 3,000 ft. elevation. Java, Tropical Africa.

Acalypha australis Linn.

A. *chinensis* Roxb.

Family: Euphorbiaceae

Slender herb up to 1 m. high; stem slender; trailing or straggling, copiously branched, green rarely purplish, hispidly hairy. Leaves simple, alternate, petiolate, petiole slender, ovate-lanceolate, crenate, acute, glabrate above, glabrous beneath, 3-nerved, 7x3 cm., stipules slender, about 1 mm. long, hairy. Flowers in erect, elongate, lax spikes, monoecious spikes about 7 cm. long, peduncles slender about 6 cm. long. Male flowers minute, clustered towards the apex, embracteate, reddish, minutely pedicelled. Perianth segments 4, free, membranous, 4-partite, ovate, concave, glabrous. Stamens 8; filaments free, very small, white, connective prolonged into a hood-like strucure above the anther. Female flowers in spikes of 1-4 bracts with a stalked solitary bract or some times at the base of large accrescent, leafy bract, low on the male spikes Carpels 3, synocarpus, green; ovary superior 3-gonous, 3-rarely, 4-celled, ovoid, lower half glabrous, upper half muricately hairy. Styles 3, about 1 mm. long, long, reddish split into 2 subulate, filiform arms. Stigmas linear, simple, free to the base, ovule solitary in each cell. Capsule with muricately bulbous based, ovoid, regma of 3-4 cocci, crustaceous, 2-valved; cocci ovoid. Seeds reddish.

Flowering and fruiting: October-December

Distribution: Native of China extending to Japan. Naturalised in India. Common in tea estates and gardens, Dehradun, Uttar Pradesh.

Acalypha australis Linn. Erect, branched, annual herbs, 30-60 cm. tall. Leaves ovate to lanceolate, with a rounded base, acute, coarsely toothed, appressed hairy, 3-8 x 1.5 - 3.5 cm. Flowers in axillary, peduncled spikes. Male and female flowers. Capsules 0.3 cm. across, pilose. Seeds ovoid, dark, brown, smooth. Female fls. in the upper part of the spike, sessile, naked.

The species *Acalypha australis* Linn. is distinguished from *Acalypha brachystachya* Hornem. on the basis of certain characters particularly *A. australis* has foliaceous, ovate-cordate, cucullate, 3-5-flowered bracts. In other species *A.*

ciliata and *A. brachystachya*, the bracts of male flowers are not foliaceous.

Acalypha lanceolata Willd.

Urtica pilosa Lour. (non *Acalypha pilosa* Cav.)

Acalypha fallax Muell. Arg.

A. wightiana Muell.-Arg.

A. boehmerioides Miquet.

A. hispida Herb.

A. virginiana Herb.

A. corchorifolia Vahl.

A. flexuosa Herb.

Family: Euphorbiaceae

Annual 6-18 in. high, usually branched from the base, flaccid or rather rigid, more or less pubescent and with sometimes long deciduous hairs on the stem. Leaves very variable, 1-4 in., membranous; petals shorter or longer than the limb. Spikes 1-5 in.; male fls. in a minute head concealed by the upper-most bracts, or produced into a minute spike; bracts always 1-fid, 9-12-toothed. Capsules hispid, styles rather short, laciniate. Seeds globosely ovoid, nearly smooth.

Flowering and fruiting:	September-November
Distribution:	Deccan Peninsula; from Mysore and the Circars southwards, common. Burma; Ceylon, common. Sumatra, Java.

Acalypha lanceolata Willd.

Annual puberulous herb 15-45 cm. high. Leaves 2.5 x 1 - 2.5 cm. long; petiole slender, 1-3 cm, long. Flowers borne in short sessile axillary or in terminal spikes; male flowers very minute in small fasicles, almost concealed by the upper most bracts or produced in a short spikes, pistillate somewhat distantly borne below the males, each in the axil of a conspicuous 8-12 toothed, persistent bract. Fruit 0.2 - 0.3 cm. across, much exerted from the bracts, cocci hispid. Seeds 0.15 cm. long, ovoid, glabrous, brown.

Plant occurring abundantly throughout the hilly forests after rains; Upper Gangetic Plains, Siwaliks.

Genus *Acalypha* Linnaeus in large genus of herbs and shrubs, comprising some 400 species, found throughout the tropics; some are cultivated in gardens for their ornamental foliage and catkins; many are wild. About nine species are found in India and a few are medicinal.

Genus *Acalypha* Linn. in the family Euphorbiaceae (about 300 genera and 3,000 species of cosmopolitan distribution, absent or very rare in arctic region) has about 450 species in tropics and subtropics comprising herbs and shrubs or trees; and about 12 species in India, chiefly in the mountains of Southern and Western India; wild, cultivated in garden and one is naturalised.

Salient features of the genus *Acalypha* Linn.-Leaves alternate, toothed or crenate, rarely entire, penniveined or 3-6 nerved. Flowers small, monoecious or occasionally dioecious, apetalous and without a disk, arranged in axillary or terminal racemes; males minute, without bracts; females 1-2, within a peduncled solitary bract, or sometimes at the base of large accrescent leafy bracts, low on the male spikes or on separate spikes.

Males flowers-Sepals 4,. valvate, more or less connate in a membranous calyx. Stamens usually 8, or many on a convex receptacle; filaments short, free; anther cells, distinct, divaricate often becoming twisted or flexuous. Pistilodes none. Female flowers - Sepals 3-4, minute, imbricate. Ovary 3-celled; styles filiform, often long and lacinate or fimbriate; ovules solitary in each cell. Fruit a capsule of 3 minute 2-

valved crustaceous cocci. Seeds subglobose, testa crustaceous, albumen fleshy, cotyledons broad and flat.

Two species of *Acalaypha* Linn. are mainly distinguished on the basis of characters in flower and fruits. For the instance, the bracts distant, shortly dentate and capsule hispid are in *Acalypha indica* Linn.; when the bracts crowded, fimbrate and glabrous capsule are in *Acalypha ciliata* Forsk.

Some species of *Acalypha* Linn. are separated for characterstics bracts primarily. Female bracts are not foliaceous in two species which are further distinguished as male bracts deeply 3-fid and fruit hairy in *Acalypha brachystachya* Hornem.; whereas these bracts are cupular, shallowly 20-dentate and fruit glabrous in *Acalypha ciliata* Forsk.

Broadly several Indian species of the genus *Acalypha* Linn. are also grouped on the basis of prime differential characters such as female bracts solitary, very large and 2-flowered are in *Acalypha dalzellii* Hook.f.; and many other species have female spikes with many bracts, for the example, in *Acalypha paniculate* Miquel., *A. fruticosa* Fosrk., *A. alnifolia* Klein., *A. indica* Linn., *A. brachystachya* Hornem., *A. malabarica* Muell.-agg., *A. fallax* Muell.-Arg. and *A. ciliata* Forsk.

Acalypha dalzelii Hook. f. is a very remarkable species which is with androgynous spike, each consisting of one female bract, and a very slender rachis with minute male flowers, and others are wholly female, and bears axillary long peduncled female bracts in the flower of plants.

The habit of *Acalypha fruticosa* Forsk. is almost similar to *A. alnifolia* Klein., but the stems and leaves beneath are glabrous, and the latter more or less glandular. Large plants apparently of this species in male flowers only, from the sea coast, have leaves 3 in. long, deeply crenate, the young only glandular beneath.

Acalypha alnifolia Kl. distinguishes from *A. capitata* by the longer petioles and deeper lobed bracts in the former species.

Acalypha fallax Muellv. Arg. in very variable plant which has atleast three extreme forms having characterstic differences in leaves, flowers and others; and their flowers and fruits are similar in all the forms or varieties.

Acalypha brachystachya Rhornem is distinguished from *Acalypha australis* Linn. mainly for the floral characters like foliaceous, ovate-cordate, cucllate and 3-5-flowered bracts found in the formers species. This plant is of exotic origin and now naturalised in India. The species *Acalypha brachystachya* Hornem. is characterstic for 3-fid female bracts which are non-foliaceous.

Acalypha wilkesiana Muell.-Arg. and *Acalypha hispida* Burm. f. are natives of Viti Island and New Britain respectively; and they are found under cultivation as garden ornamentals of shrubby species with variegated leaves. *Acalypha wilkesiana* Muell.-Arg. may be recognized by white or greenish white or pale-red styles, inflorescences being shorter than the leaves, and 5 to 13-dentate or lobed female bracts. Other species *A. hispida* is recognized by crimson styles, inflorescence being longer than the leaves and minute and entire female bracts.

Acalypha wilkesiana Muell.-Arg. is shrubby plant with leaves usually broad, cordate, short acuminate, crenate, variously mottled with shades of red and purple; spikes slender 20 cm. or more in length, in faciniating, drooping festoons, flowers small, bright red. It is a common garden favourite species which is planted for hedges and fences around gardens and parks. Besides the two varieties *A. wilkesiana* var *marginata* T. Moore. and *A. wilkesiana* var. *macrophylla* N Taylor.

Genus *Acalypha* Linn. is mostly of herbs or shruby plants with venetation palmate, leaves serrate and ovate, pubescence and simple. In regard to important genera in the Upper Gangetic plains and Siwaliks, the genus *Acalypha* comes in group of genera and plants flowers which are not arranged in çyathia; perianth dichamydeous; ovary-cells 2-ovuled, fruit usually 3-seeded or less by abortion; perianth-segments valvate in bud, petiole without glands and stamens free and anther 4-celled.

The genus *Acalypha* Linn. falles under series II with cells or ovary-ouled, in the tribe V Crotoneae and its subtribe 4 Acalypheae with filaments free, anthers erect, 2-celled, cells united by their base only, and this genus is specific for the characters such as style very long fimbriate or lacerate, female fls. in large bracts.

The leaves, roots, flowers and whole plant of various species of *Acalypha* Linn. are medicinally useful.

The leaves of *Acalypha fruticosa* Forsk. are stomachic and useful in dyspepsia, alterative and attenuant.

Leaves of the plant are esteemed much by the users of herbal medicines recommending them as a good stomachic in dyspeptic affections and in cholera; and they are also using this plant leaves as attenuant and alterative medicine in needful conditions or correct the habit. Leaves may be used in the form of infusion in the dose of half tea-cupful twice in a day or suitable to ailing conditions and patients.

The leaves and flowers of the plant *Acalypha hispida* Burm. f. are medicinally useful in various ailments.

Flowers are considered specific for use against diarrhoea, and other similar complaints and troubles of indigestion.

Leaves are ground with green tobacco leaves and influsion of rice applied to inveterate ulcers.

Whole plant, leaves and roots of *Acalypha paniculata* Miq. ae medicinally useful, and suggested to medicinal purposes as *A. indica* Linn.

The leaves, roots stalks, young shoots and whole plant of *Acalypha indica* Linn. are medicinally useful.

Plant contains an alkaloid 'acalyphin', a cyanogenetic glucoside and triacetanamine, possibly a degradation product of the former. The glucoside crystallises in two forms, thin hexagonal plates (m.p., 182-4°) and fine silky needles (m.p., 108°). The HCN content is 270 mg. per 100 g.

In addition to HCN, the plant contains other substances which cause intense, dark chocolate-brown discoloration of blood, and gastro-intestinal irritation in rabbits, and considered extremely poisonous to them.

Chemistry of plant find that Benzene extract of the whole plant left a gummy residue which was dossolved in ether and extracted with 3 per cent NaOH solution. Ether layer was washed with water and dried, the resultant dark green gummy residue was chromatographical and eluted with petroleum ether and benzene (1:1). This yielded a fraction which on crystallisation gave a solid with m.p. 85-86°. Further elution with benzene and ether (2:1) yielded a second fraction which on further purification gave a solid m.p. 134-136°. This solid was acetylated with acetic anhydride and pyridine.

The whole plant is anthelmintic, expectorant, emetic, anodyne and hypnotic. Roots are cathartic, leaves are laxative and used in scabies and snake-bite.

According to the B.P.C., the fresh or dry plant is a gastro-intestinal irritant and has been used as a substitute for ipecacuanha. A decoction of the entire plant in doses of 1.5 - 1 oz. is used as a safe and speedy laxative. In cases of constipation in children, the bruised leaves, introduced in the manner of a suppository, invariably give relief. The juice of fresh leaves is a reliable emetic and has been found useful in cases of croup.

Leaves of the plant, ground with common salt, quick lime or lime juice is reputed to be a parasiticide and is applied externally. A paste of the leaves with lime juice is considered benefecial in early cases of ringworm but has no effect in chronic cases. Plant is quite ineffective as an anthelmintic.

The plant *Acalypha paniculata* Miq. is sometimes used as a substitute for *Acalypha indica* Linn.

This plant is growing as a troublesome weed in gardens and roadsides and other various places throughout the plains of country and commonly available for collection and usage for medicinal purposes as remedy against different ailments.

The roots, tender shoots and leaves are employed in various medicinal recipes given in several complaints.

The powder of the dry leaves is considered useful for giving to children suffering from worm affections. Besides the decoction is prepared from the leaves by addition of garlic which is also useful in worms a complaints. The juice of the whole plant specially leaves, together with that of the tender shoots, is occasionally mixed with a small portion of margosa oil, rubbed on the tongue of infants for the purpose of sickening them and clearing their stomachs of viscid phlegm.

The leaves with garlic are regarded as anthelmintic; mixed with common salt the leaves are applied externally in the skin affections like scabies, erruptions and itching. The juice is rubbed up with oil is used externally in rheumatism. The plant is considered useful in consumption.

The roots are regarded as purgative medicine and for this purpose, the juice or decoction is used in constipation. The roots and leaves are frequently used as laxative herbal and considered useful for abdomen and the organs of digestive system due to their effect as stomachic, anthelminitic, purgative, aromatic, stimulant and carminative.

The plant has also reputation of an expectorant and used in cough and asthma and respiratory ailments including throat, lungs and chest complaints. Its one of the native names as Khakli means to cough relevantly.

The expressed juice of the plant is much regarded wherever growing, as an emetic medicine for children, and considered safe, certain and speedy in its action.

Like the official drug Ipecacuanha, it seems to have little tendency to act on the bowels or to depress the vital powers, and it decidedly increases the secretion of the pulmonary organs. Probably an infusion of the dried leaves or an extract prepared from the green plant, would retain all its active properties. For this purpose, the leaves juice may be given one or half teaspoonful medicine to infants and also to other patients of higher are groups, with necessary addition.

The decoction of leaves is given in earache; a cataplasm of the leaves is applied as a local application to syphilitic ulcers, and as a means of relieving the pain of snake-bite.

The roots of the plant attract cats quite as much as those of valerian. Plant is considered useful in cases of acute mania. The fresh juice with chloride of sodium dissolved in it and dropped in both nostrils every morning, followed by cold shower-baths for three mornings regularly, proves highly successful. Thus it is supposed by them to act as a 'brain purge', so called probably owing to a quantity of mucus and other matter escaping from the nostrils immediately after the application of the above recipe. It is given internally to act as an anthelmintic and laxative.

The juice of the fresh leaves mixed with lime is applied topically in painful rheumatic affections. It is used in scabies and ringworm, also internally as a carminative.

The roots possess purgative properties; the leafjuice is a safe and useful emetic, especially adapted for children.

The juice of the fresh plant is considered useful in children and given as an emetic in child dose or small quantity. It is suggested for emesis purpose in ailing conditions in children. The plant carries a native name as Chalmari in Kanara and also Kuppi which means to a heap; and it is relevant to the habitat of plant as this plant grows frequently in waste places and rubbish heaps. From these localities the plant is procured for medicinal uses.

This herb is used in congestive headaches. A piece of cotton is saturated with the expressed juice and inserted into each nostril, relieving the head symptoms by causing haemorrhage from the nose. The powder of the dry leaves is used in bed sores ad wounds attacked by worms.

The whole plant or leaves are considered useful in conditions of asthma and bronchitis, and this herbal remedy is given both in children and adults.

A herbal recipe was made of this plant. The mode of preparation is that macerate 3 oz. of the fresh leaves, stalks and flowers with a pint (or 473 cc. -20 fluid oz.) of spirits or wine, in the closed jar for 7 days, occasionally agitating the mixture. Strain, press, filter and add sufficient spirits of ether to make or pint. Physiological effects of this formula are indicated that in small doses it is expectorant and nauseant in large doses emetic. In posological consideration, the doses of minims (or drops) 20 to 60, frequently repeated during the day in honey.

One drachm (or 60 minims) of the expressed juice of the fresh leaves of plant is an easy and rapid emetic in childred. A few drops or minis may be suggested for low-age infants or in higher doses for grown up children. It may be useful as expectorant aginst cough or chest complaints and cough ailments, and also in other ailing conditions needy of emesis.

The leaves of the plant *Acalypha alnifolia* Klein ex Willd. are medicinally useful. Leaves juice or infusion is given in dysentery.

Whole plant, leaves and roots of *Acalypha ciliata* Forsk. are medicinally useful. Leaves paste is applied to ulcers. Whole plant is used in bronchitis, asthma, pneumonia and rheumatism, and also other similar complaints.

The bruised leaves of *Acalypha indica* Linn. are suggested to be useful as an application to maggot-eaten sores.

The roots, well bruished in hot water, are recommended as a cathartic, and the leaves as a laxative in decoction mixed with common salt.

The leaves are used in scabies, and mixed with chunam in other cutaneous diseases. Medicinal properties and actions of the plant drug-Rasa Tikta-kaṣāya, Virya uṣṇa, Vipāka kaṭu, Guna uṣṇa, Vāta-kapha nāsaka, pittasaṁsamana (or tridoṣahara); Karma dīpana, pācana, sāṅgrāhi, tvacya, kaṇḍūghna, sleṣmanihsāraka, viṣaghna, sāraka, vāmaka, kramighna, recaka, uttejaka, kāsa ghna, saumanasyajanana, raktarodhaka vraṇaropaṇa and vedanāsthāpana.

Therapeutic indications or āmayika prayoga as external and internal uses in various Roga or disease-kāsa, svāsa, vibandha, bāla-roga (kāsa, udaravikāra and in vamana-recana karma), viṣa, āmavāta, vātavyādhi, atisāra, pravāhikā, urahvikāra, vraṇa-krimi, tvacavikara or carmaroga-dadru-pāmākaṇḍū, vraṇa, mānasavikāra and other vikāra.

Haritamañjarī, the Sanskrit name for plant drug.

2

Agave cantula Roxb.

A. wightii non.rain

Agave americana auct. L.

A. mexicana

A. cantala Roxb.

Family: Agavaceae

Regional names: Maguey, Cantala, Bombay Aloe (English), Kalnaru (Kannar), Ghayal (Marathi)

Perennial, somewhat stout, scapigerous herbs. Stems very short, woody, simple, with a crown of rosette leaves. Leaves patent, recurved in the upper part, remotely apinescently dentate with upwardly hooked spines, with a 1·2 cm. long, sharp, dark brown anine of the acicular tip, up to 150 x 8-10 cm. Scapes stout, scaly, up to 3-5 m. tall, patently branched at the top. Flowers greenish, in panicles. Pedicles jointed, 0.8-1 cm. long. Tepals lanceolate, with obtuse, ligulate tips; inner ones smaller and narrower than the outer ones. Stamens exerted; filaments brown-blotc̃hed. 6-7.5 cm. long; anthers 3-3.5 cm. long. Style 6.5-8 cm. long. Bulbils present.

Flowering and fruiting: July-September

Plant occurring in the Upper Gangetic Plains, Siwaliks; in waste places, roadsides, often planted along hedges and borders of field; northern India, and various other areas in the country.

Naturalised in many parts of India, extending from central India to both Eastern and Western coasts to the North-East Gangetic Plains and to the sub-Himalayan tracts.

Agave wightii Drumm.

A. wightii Drummond & Prain.

A. angustifoia Haworth.

Agave vivipara Wight.

A. cantula Dalz. & Gibs. (non. Roxb.)

Family: Agavaceae

Regional names: Banskeora

Perennial somewhat stout herbs. Stems woody, simple, with a rosette of leaves, upto 30-45 cm. high. Leaves erect, narrowed at both ends, constricted at base, with a spinescently dentate margins, and an apiculate tip with a 1-2 cm. long, dark brown spine, 45-70 x 7-10 cm. Spines stout, upcurved. Scapes stout, scaly, 2-4 m. high. Flowers in terminal panicles. Pedicels, 1.5-2 cm. long. Tepals lanceolate obtuse. Stamens 6; filaments sub-equal, linear, 5-6 cm. long, exerted. Anthers 2 cm. long. Style 5 cm. long. Stigma 3-lobed. Bulbils present.

A plant with stout trunk and a stiff, compact rosette of leaves about 2 ft. long add 3 inch. broad at the middle, and with weak marginal prickles.

Flowering and fruiting: July-September

It is naturalised in the sub-Himalayan tract and outer Himalayan and many other parts of India. In the plains, it is grown as a fence along railway lines.

Agave wightii Drum. & Pr. syn. *A. augustifolia* How. Plant with stout trun, usually conspicuous. Leaves ensiform, linear-lanceolate, up to 100 x 10 cm., many, forming a stiff rosette; marginal prickles spreading or erect, with a small, brown cushion, sharply recurved and parallel to the leaf edge; terminal spine pale, decurrent.

Plant commonly found in waste places, roadsides, forest clearings; and often planted along hedges or bunds of the gardens, and many other places in the regions of occurrence in different parts of country.

It is one of the commonest species generally found in the Himalayan regions. Plant *Agave angustifolia* Haw. is specific with grey-green leaves with a black terminal spine, and marginal black-brown teeth. Sometimes it is not easily distinguished by the planters from *A. amaericana* Linn.

Agave wightii D. & P.; Small aloe of India. The plant is cultivated and naturalised in the Upper Gangetic Plains, Siwaliks, Rohilkhand, Terai, and from Delhi or Haryana southwards to Ludhiana, Punjab.

It is the only *Agave* species in northern India which develops a conspicuous trunk. Its native country is not known. A variegated form is often cultivated in gardens. This plant holds definitely its own place as a hedge plant, especially in the drier provinces. Naturalised in many parts of India. It is found in Burma. Its native country is not known for certain. This appears to be the first *Agave* species to reach India, and it came prbably from the Pacific coast of Central America. The fibre exported from Bombay with that of other species is often wrongly identified *Agave vivioera.* The freshly cut leaves smell like rhubarb.

Leaves linear-lanceolate pale-green or sometimes glabrous, very narrow in proportion to their length 4ft. or more, the greatest width just above the middle being about 3 in., curving onwards gradually from their bases or bent over almost from their origin; upper surface portion; marginal petioles large; alcate always ascending. 1/4 in. or more long, very sharp, pale-brown or garmet-coloured, from a small light coloured cushion; terminal spine acicular, cylindrical, reddish or dark brown 1/2 in. long.

Agave americana Linn.

Regional names: Kantala (Hindi), Jungli anaras (Bengla), Wiliyatthaitalu (Punjabi), Alagai (Tamil), Kittanara (Telgu)

Rakas-pattah, bans-keora, bara kanwar, hathi-sengar, ram kanta, hathi chinghar (Hindi), Jungli or bilati-ananash, anards bans-keora, bilaipat, koyan (Bengla), Seubbara (Arabic), Parkand (Marathi), Rakas-patta (Deccan), Jangli-kunvara (Gujrati), Pitha kalabuntha (Tamil), Rakashimatalu (Telgu), Panam-kairasha (Malayalam). The Century Plant, The American Aloe, The Carata (English); Pita or Magury (Spain).

Stemless plant. Leaves erecto-patent, with strong, widely patent or recurved marginal spines, glaucous, often with longitudinal, white or yellow streaks or bands; larger ones with recurved upper halves. Perianth funnel-shaped; segments oblong, yellowish green. Capsule oblong-clavate, beaked.

Trunk prostrate or ascending; leaves deep-green often variegated with white or pale-yellow stripes or borders, sometimes rather glabrous; marginal prickles mostly pointing downwards; terminal spine dull-brown, 1-2 in. long; perianth lobes obtuse, amber-coloured.

The American Aole plant is planted in parks and large gardens throughout India, but not naturalised. Cultivated, often met with as an escape in waste places.

Outside India, it is cultivated as an ornamental plant in gardens in North Europe and North America. The plant widely naturalised and commonly termed as *Agave americana* is South Europe is believed to be *A. vera-crux* Miller.

The plant *Agave americana* Linn. is originally a native of America: and naturalised in some or many parts of India gradually, but nowhere occurs gregariously while plentiful throughout the country. Planted in parks and large gardens, grown along railway lines, and in many other parts of hotter regions in country.

Agave vera-cruz Mill. The Blue Elephant Aloe Plant with leaves linear-oblong, recurved of drooping, glaucous.

Cultivated, often met with as an escape in the waste place in various areas. Naturalised throughout India; common in Assam, Bengal, Bihar, Bombay and South India.

Plant commoner in the upper than in lower India, specially in the North-West Provinces, almost not common in Bengal.

The plant raises its cluster of leaves upon a short, erect stem, which produces vivaparous buds. It is all together a much less robust plant. The leaves are less fleshy and erect instead of reflexed. The flowering stem is not more than half the height of that of *Agave americana*, and much thinner and red-coloured. In the lacalities where they grow side by side they appear (both plants) quite distinct.

Genus *Agave* in the family Agavaceae Endl. or Sisal Family, sometimes included under family Amaryllidaceae (sens. lat.).

Agave Linneaus in family Agavaceae (20 genera and 670 species in tropics and subtropics; 4 genera and 15 species in India, mostly in hotter parts) has about 300 species distributed from Southern United States to tropical South America; and 6 species naturalised and cultivated in different parts of India.

Genus *Agave* Linn. with salient features-Stem short, thick. leaves radical, fleshy, usually spiny. Inflorescence large, usually paniculate. Perinanth connate at base, segments, narrow and erect, shorter than stamens. Staminal filaments filiform, not flattened. Ovary inferior; ovules many, biseriate; style filiform, stigma subcapitate.

Various genera found in India have distinguishing characters in Agavaceae family. Ovary inferior, flowers in panicles and perianth gamophyllous in the genus *Agave* Linn.; whereas the genera *Furcraea* Vent. differs by perianth polyphyllous; and genus *Polianthes* Linn. has inferior ovary and flowers in simple spikes. Leaves armed, at least with terminal thorn, peduncle more than 4 m., ovary inferior, flowers large, over 10 cm. long; tepals erect, much exceeded by stamens and style are specific characters in genus *Agave* Linn.

Plant is recognizable by ensiform leaves, linear-lanceolate, very many, 2.5-3 ft. long, and up to 3.5 in. at its widest part, inserted in a compact series on a stout usually consipicuous trunk which is partly procumbent or throughout ascending, forming a stiff even rosette 3-5 ft. in diam. pale-green or often tinged with ashy grey, base thin, broadly amplexicaule; marginal prickles rather weak, about 3/4 in. apart, usually consisting of a small brown cushion carrying a semi-transparent garnet-coloured spine which is often sharply recurved parallel to the leaf edge, but ending in a finely barbed hook pointing upwards; terminal spine about 1/2 in. long, pale, slightly decurrent.

Agave sisalana Perrine ex Engelm.

Family: Agavaceae

Regional names: The Sisal Hemp, the (English). Henequrn Fibre or Sisal Hemp of America

Plant with leaves linear-lanceolate, pruinose. Perianth 5-6 cm. long (including ovary); segments oblong, with a tuft of hairs on the inner side at the top; upper half of the segments soon marcescent with inrolled margins, finally reflexed. Bulbils present.

Agave sisalana Perrine ex Engelm. Leaves with smallish spines along margins, up to 200 x 16 cm. ashy grey, fleshy. Inflorescence paniculate, 4-6 m. tall, to 25 cm. thick at the base. Perianth white, 2-4 cm. long. Stamens 6 cm. long. Ovary 3-4 cm. long.

Flowering and fruiting: All seasons

Native to Neotropics. Common in upper Ghats and across plains. Planted as hedge or for fiber.

Cultivated, often met with as an escape in waste places It is cultivated in many parts of India as far North in Punjab and Lahore in Pakistan, also in Central India, Bombay, Bengal, Mysore and Madras, and also in Burma and other adjacent regions. It is also grown in Australia, Fiji, Hawai and East Africa. In the beginning, the sisal hemp was known in Yucatan and then it was introduced to Florida and there naturalised; and from Florida it was brought to the West India Islands and thence to India.

Various species of the genus *Agave* Linn. are distinguishable by characters of leaves, spines and flowers. Leaves with horny margins or provided with minute spines are specific in *Agave sisalana* Perrr. & Engeim.; whereas some other species generally have leaves with distinct coarse marginal spines. Further they (species) are separated for characterstic spines, as spines of leaf-margins patent or obliquely deflexed, with upcurved tips are in two species *Agave americana* Linn. and *A. vera-cruz* Mill. which are distinct of leaf-characters such as oblong-lanceolate leaves contracted into a collar above the base are in *Agave americana* Linn. when *A. vera-cruz* Mill. is with liner-oblong leaves which are not contracted into a collar. Other two species *Agave wightii* Drumm & Prain and *A. cantala* Roxb. are with spines of leaf-margins erecto-patent, with tips curved towards the leaf-apex. Further these species are distinguishable of flower characters as tepals free near to the base or connate at base only, and flowers up to 4-4.5 cm. long are in *Agave wightii* D. & P.; whereas tepals connate in the lower part, and flowers 7-8 cm. long in *A. cantala* Roxb. length of leaves may also çomparatively differ in two species as leaves up to 100 cm. long in *Agave wightii* D. & P. and leaves exceed upto 150-200 cm. long in *A. cantala* Roxb.

Two major genera of Agavaceae primarily differ for leaves characters. Genus *Agave* Linn. or Century plants has leaves usually spine-edged, whereas the leaves mostly entire in genus *Yucca* Linn. Leaves in a very large basal rosette, narrow-lanceolate spine-tipped and often a spiny margins, in *Agave* Linn.

The roots, leaves and gums of *Agave americana* Linn. are medicinally useful.

The roots are diuretic and anti-syphilitic. Sap is laxative, diuretic, emmenagogue and antiscorbutic.

Hecogenin was obtained in a greater yield from the residues left after extraction of long fibres (sisal fibres) from *A. cantala.* The petroleum ether extract on removal of the solvent yielded the sapogenin residue which, on purification by chromatography, yielded pure hecogenin m.p. 260°-265°, and gave hecogenin acetate m.p. 243°-245°, and hecogenin benzoate m.p. 260°.

Hecogenin was also isolated from the leaves of *Agave americana* in a yield of 0.065 per cent. Its idenity was confirmed by mixed melting point determination.

Chlorogenin was isolated in a yield of 0.3 per cent from the fresh flowers of *Agave americana.* The flavonol glycoside were identified as kaempferol-3-glucoside and kaempferol-3-rutinocide.

Pharmacological studies find that Polyfructosan obtained from *Agave vera-cruz* and inulin at 5 per cent levels, fed to rats for a period of 6 weeks reduced cholosterol levels in plasma very significantly, while in liver there was no reduction of cholesterol level except in insulin fed rats which were given exagenous cholesterol. A slight increase in the faecal excretion of sterols (digitonin precipitate) was observed in rats fed with polyfructosan while with inulin no difference was observed.

The roots, leaves and whole plant of *Agave americana* Linn. are medicinally useful.

Roots are diuretic, diaphoretic and antisyphilitic. Juice of leaves is useful as laxative, diuretic, emmenagogue, and in scurvy. Whole plant is fish poison.

Plant contains saponins; and leaves contain saponin.

The roots and leaves of *Agava angustifolia* Haw. are medicinally useful.

Roots are diuretic and diaphoretic. Juice of leaves is applied to bruises.

The plant *Agave vera-cruz* Mill. is medicinally useful. Plant is purgative.

The large, moist and fleshy leaves of *Agave americana* Linn. are sometimes used as a poultice. The roots are said to find their way to Europe mixed with Sarsaparilla. In Mexican uses of plant, the roots afford a palatable and nutritious food when properly cooked.

The expressed juice of the leaves is administered as a resolvent and alterative, especially in syphilis.

The leaves, as also the roots when cut, yield a saccharine juice which by evaporation may be converted into a syrup having a peculiar nauseous odour and acid taste; it reddens litmus paper. This is administered, having attributed to it resolvent and alterative properties; it is regarded as specially useful in syphilis. The roots are said to have employed in secondary syphilis with great apparent benefit in the form of decoction, in the proportion of four ones to one pint of water.

The marine cordage the fibre compares favourably in durability with Manila hemp. It has also been used for the manufacture of coarse fabrics. It is commonly used for binders, twine, fishing nets, hammocks, door mats, rugs, carpets etc. The refuge left after decorticating the leaves is employed in making paper and paper-boards.

A large quantity of juice is obtained from *Agave americana* Linn. (Century plant or American Aloe), when fermented, it yields pulque, the national drink of Mexico, the distiiled spirit is known as meseal.

It is stated that Agaves popularly called the Century plants. After flowering and seeding the plant dies, but from the ground daughter off-shoots spring up, and thus a hedgerow of Agave continues to flower year after year.

Kaṇṭāla, the Sanskrit name for plant drug.

The sap is stated to be laxative, diuretic and emmenagogue, and in dose of two fluid ounces, three times a day, has been found very useful in scurvy, and as a great success in scurvy. The disagreable smell of the juice, which has been compared to that of putrid meat, causes a person at first to turn from it in disgust, but after a while the odour is overcome, and liking for it takes the place of the previous dislike.

The large, moist and fleshy leaves are stated to have been used with much advantage, as a poultice; the fresh juice is applied to bruises and contusions.

The gum found exuding from the leaves and lower part of the stem is used as a cure for toothache.

The pulp of the leaves placed between folds of muslin is applied to the eye in conjunctivitis; it is also used, mixed with sugar, in gonorrhoea twice a day. Medicinal properties and action of plant drug-Rosa tikta-kaṭu-kaṣāya, Vipaka katu, Virya usna, Vātapitta sāmaka (tridoṣasāmaka), Guna laghu; and Karma sāraka, vraṇaropaṇa, mūtrala, svedajanana, raktaskandana, raktaprasādana, balya, racikara, cakṣuṣya, dantya, tvadya, sothahara, stambhana, nāḍībalya and kṛmighna.

Therapeutic indication in vraṇa, vraṇasotha, kaṣata, arsa-aṅkura, jalodara, sotha, atisara, phiraṅga, upadaṁsa, youna-vikāra (sambhogajanya), dantasūla, netravikāra, pravāhikā, mūtravikāra, jvara, agnidagdha and other various ailments. Kaṇṭāla, Kumāripatra and Sūtravarā, the Sanskrit names for plant drug.

In cultivation pattern several species become variegated in colour, the most striking being one with golden bands along the leaves. They take several years to reach the flowering stage, and from the fact that in adverse circumstances their development may be retarded from 10 to 50 or 100 years, they are popularly called the Century plants. After flowering and seeding the plant dies, but from the ground daughter off-shoots spring up, and thus a hedgerow of Agave continues to flower year after year.

Kantala, the Sanskrit name for plant drug.

The sap is stated to be laxative, diuretic and emmenagogue, and in dose of two fluid ounces, three times a day, has been found very useful in scurvy. The great success in scurvy. The disagreable smell of the juice, which has been compared to that of putrid meat, causes a person at first to turn from it in disgust, but after a while the odour is overcome, and liking for it takes the place of the previous dislike.

The large, moist and fleshy leaves are stated to have been used with much advantage, as a poultice; the fresh juice is applied to bruises and contusions.

The gum found exuding from the leaves and lower part of the stem is used as a cure for toothache.

The pulp of the leaves placed between folds of muslin is applied to the eye in conjunctivitis; it is also used, mixed with sugar, in gonorrhoea twice a day.

The roots are diuretic; and used by the natives in chronic gonorrhoea.

The juice of *Agave vivpara* L., alongwith the flower of *Eleusine curacana,* is applied to contusions of draught-cattles.

The plant *Agave saponaria* is a powerful detergent; its roots are used as a substitute for soap.The sap has detergent properties.

The leaves, roots, and plant of *Agave cantula* Roxb. syn. *Agave americanum* auct. non L. are medicinally useful.

The plant is useful in anasarca, ascites, dropsy, dysentery, syphilis, veneral diseases and other similar complaints.

The roots are useful as anthelmintic, and is paralysis, fever goitre, skin diaseses and diarrhoea.

The leaves are useful in boils, burn, cuts, wounds, skin diseases and warts.

The leaves are useful in veterinary diseases.

The leaves of Agaves yield a valuable fibre. *Agave sisalana* is source of the wellknown sisal fibre. *Agave vera-cruz, A. heteracantha* Zucc. and *A. lecheguilla* Torr. yield fibres of inferior quality. Agave fibre is one of the imprtant hard fibres. Agave fibre is mostly used for making ropes, cordage and twine. The shorter fibres and istles are used for making mops and brushes. Sisal is eminently suited for cordage of all kinds of trials carried out that for.

Marine Cordage, the fibre compares favourably in durability with Manila hemp.

3

Ajuga bracteosa Wall. ex Benth.

Ajuga remota Benth.

Ajuga bracteosa Wall.

Family: Lamiaceae (Labiatae)

Regional names: Kauri-buti (Jhelum), Karku, Nilkanthi (Sutlej), Khurauri (Trans-Indus Punjab); Ratpatha, Rat-patiya, Neel-kanthi; Jan-inadam; Mukund babri (Punjab and Noth-West provices); Janiddam

Erect-ascending often caespitose, branches from the base, pubescent villous, perennial herbls, with a woody base. Lower leaves long-petioled; upper ones sessile; all leaves oblanceolate-obovate, with a narrowed base, obtuse or rounded cren ate-dentate, appressed-hairy above, densely appressed, pubescent beneath, 1.5-15 x 1-3 cm. Flowers subsessile. Calyx 0.5 - 0.6 cm. long, glandular-villous outside. Corolla blue or pink, hairy outside, 0.8-1 cm. long Stamens exerted. Nutlets ovoid-ellipsoid, reticulate, 0.25 x 0.13-0.15 cm.

Flowering and fruiting: January-December

Plant occurring common in grassy, sandy localities of river-beds, roadsides and forest clearings in Siwaliks, Dehradun and adjoining areas in region.

Ajuga ramota Benth. syn. *Ajuga bracteosa* Wall.

An ascending with herb. Stem diffusely branching from the base. Leaves ovate, lower ones stalked, upper sessile.

Flowers pale blue, crowded in axillary whorls forming leafy spikes more or less interrupted near the base. Corolla tube 2 times or long as the calyx.

Flowering in April to October.

Throughout north India, ascending 2300 m. alt.; Kumaon region, U.P. hills ascending to 2300 m. alt.

Ajuga bracteosa Wallich ex Bentham

Flowers pale blue to whitish, with corolla-tube nearly twice as long as clayx, 2-lipped with upper lip very short 2-lipped the lower lip 3-lobed; borne in crowded whorls forming leafy spike-like clusters. Corolla c. 1 cm. calyx densely hairy; bracts often blue, ovate to elliptic, coarsely toothed, overlapping, longer than the flowers. Leaves 2.5-3 cm., oblanceolate blunt, wavy-toothed, hairy, the lower short, the upper stalkless; stems many spreading, leafy, hairy, 10-30.

Distribution: Afganistan to Bhutan, India, China, Japan, South-east Asia, from 1000 to 4000 m. alt., in open slopes, commonly growing with flowering during the period from June to September

Ajuga bracteosa Wall. syn. *Ajuga ramota* Benth.

Stems or branches many from the rootstock, 4-12 in., simple or divided, usually stout, leafy, pubescent most variable. Leaves 1-4 in., lower petioled, upper sessile. Calyx 1/4 in., villous, teeth half the length of the tube, ovate-lanceolate, acute. Corolla pale blue or lilac, pubescent; tube rarely twice as long as the calyx; upper lip erect 2-fid; side lobes of lower oblong, midlobe dilated variable in length. Nutlets ellipsoid, deeply rugosely pitted.

A. bracteosa Wall. var. *densiflora.* Stem scapiform, radical leaves obovate-oblong obtuse subentive, cauline O or oblong sessile; spike 2-3 in. villous; bracts shorter than the flower, corolla very shortly exerted.

A. densiflora Wall.-Nepal. It appears like a starved *A. bracteosa,* which the form of the calyx, corolla and nutlets entirely resembling. *Ajuga ramota* Benth. is not separable from *A. bracteosa,* which are probably intended to include the form with distant whorls and large floral leaves.

Distribution: Western Himalaya, from Kashmir to Nepal, alt. 1000-7000 ft. elevation, and in the plains near them from Oudh to Peshawar. Afghanistan, China, Japan, Abysina.

Ajuga bracteosa Wall.

Perennial herb. softly hairy or glabrate, stolons none; branches many, 4-12 in. long, usually stout, erect or ascending, simple or branching, leafy. Leaves 1-4 in. long, ovate oblanceolate or subspathulate obtuse, sinuate-toothed, the lower petioled. Whorls axillary, often crowded in spikes. Flowers 1/4-1/3 in. long; bracts leaf-like, longer than the whorls, ovate or cuneate-obovate, entire or toothed. Calyx 1/8 in.long, villous. Corolla pale-blue or lilac. Stamens exerted. Nutlets 1/10 in long, deeply rugose.

Plant occuring in Siwalik range foothills, Terai and eastwards in the Sub-Himalayan tracts of Rohilkhand and North Oudh. Western Himalayan region from Kashmir to Nepal (upto 7,000 ft. elevation) and on the Punjab plains along the base of hills from Peshawar.

Ajuga macrosperma Wall. ex Benth.

Ajuga repens Roxb.

Ajuga geniculata Maxim.

Family: Lamiaceae (Labiatae)

Regional names: Nandunghar

Stems or branches 6 in. to 3 ft., sometimes as thick as a swan's quill, spreading and branching, sometimes rooting, and glabrous or densely pubescent or villous. Leaves 1-6 in. long, very variable in breadth, narrowed into the often very long petiole, rarely lobed or cut. Spikes 1-8 in., whorls continuous or interrupted, lower bracts leaf-like. Calyx short, teeth always obtuse. Corolla acute, tube twice as long as the calyx, usually glabrous, limb small; upper lip, erect, 2-lobed; lobes of lower subequal or mid lobe broadest. Nutlets deeply rugosely pitted.

Ajuga macrosperma var. *thomson* Maxim. Glaborus, stems slender flaccid rooting prostrate, spikes with a very slender rachis, calyx-teeth very short rounded, corolla glabrous, tube. exerted.

Eastern Himalaya, Sikkim (6,000-9,000 ft. alt. elevation). *Ajuga macrosperma* var. *breviflora.* Smaller, branches more slender than the type 4 in-2 ft., corolla-tube shorter sometimes quite included often hairy.

Ajuga decumbens Dun., *A. sikkimensis* Miq.- Higher parts of the Khasia Mts., ascending to 10,000 ft. alt. in Sikkim.

All the Himalayan forms of *A. macropserma* perhaps may refer to this species.

Ajuga macrosperma Wall. is very variable. In the higher elevations, it assumes a lower and more slender form with smaller leaves as in *A. sikkimensis* Miq., with the corolla laxly and the tube scarcely exerted. The form has sometimes stems only a few inches high and irregularly leaves. Generally Japanese Ajuga has not with geniculate corolla-tube. *Ajuga decumbens* Maximovicx differs in the deeper calyx-lobes, the more prominent midlobe of the corolla, and in the minutely upland state of *A. thomsoni* is certainly only an upland state of *A. macropserma*; however, unlike the extreme low-land form, it is united by intermediates collected around lower regions. In general, *A. macrosperma* is a very common species in the hilly regions of northern India, being the largest of the genus, in the low grounds forming a bushy herb or sometimes 3 ft. high, with widely spreading decumbent branches and abundant spikes of blue flowers.

Ajuga macrosperma Wall ex. Benth.

Erect, ascending or clambering from the decumbent creeping base, annual herbs. Stems densely villus with long, whitish hairs towards the apex, thinly pilose, downwards. Leaves on 1.5-5 cm. long petioles elliptic-ovate to oblong-obovate, with a narrowed base, obtuse or rather acute, serrate-dentate, thinly pilose, 4-15x2-6 cm. Flowers on 0.15-0.3 cm. long, pedicels. Calyx 0.4-0.4 cm. long. Corolla blue, hairy without, 0.7-0.8 cm. long. Stamens exerted. Nutlets oblong, reticulate-rugose, 0.18-0.19 (-0.2) cm. long.

Plant occurring commonly in humid, shaded lacilities of ravines and riversides; Siwaliks, Dehradun add adjoining regions, hilly areas, Uttar Pradesh. Flowering during February to June or winter-end to summers usually.

Ajuga macrosperma Wall. ex Benth. syn. *A. repens* Roxb. A decumbent or prostrate herb, glabrous or some what pubescent. Stems or branches 1/2-3 ft., often stout, spreading and branching and sometimes rooting from the nodes, glabrous or densely hairy. Leaves stalked, 2-6 in. long variable in breadth, ovate-oblong or obovate, obtuse, sinute-crenate, rarely lobed or cut, narrowed into the often very long petiole. Whorls continuous or interrupted; lower bracts leaf-like; upper ovate, shorter than the calyx. Calyx-teeth very short obtuse. Corolla blue, usually glabrous; tube twice as long as the calyx, inflated at the base, geniculate above the swelling; limb small, upper lip erect, lobes of lower lip, subequal or the midlobe broader. Stamens exerted. Nutlets 1/18-1/20 in. rugosely pitted.

Plant occurring in sub-tropical and temperate Himalayas from Kumaon to Bhutan, upto 8000 ft. Khasia mountains and Chittagong, extending to Burma and China. Siwaliks,

Dehradun and other areas, Uttar Pradesh hilly region, and eastwards along the Sub-Himalayan tracts of Rohilkhand, North Oudh and Gorakhpur and adjoining areas. Flowering in the period from March to April. Eastern Himalayan region, Khasia mts. and Chittagong, extending to Burma and China.

Ajuga lupulina Maxim.

Densely hairy perennial with white flowers with mauve markings and with a pale blue tube, borne in whorls aggregated into a dense ovoid spike, with long overlapping pale bracts spreading much beyond the flowers. Corolla c. 1 cm., lower lip with bi-lobed central lobe and 2 rather small or lateral lobes; calyx hairy; bracts ovate-lanceolate to 3 cm., often conspicuously net-veined. Leaves obovate, stalked, coarsely toothed, upto 10 cm., stems densely woolly hairly, erect 10-25 cm.

Flowering and fruiting: June-July

Distribution: Western and Central Nepal, Tibet, 2800-4300 m., Open slopes, commonly growing in the region.

Ajuga lobata D. Don.

Flowers lilac, c. 1.5 cm., with corolla-tube nearly three times as long as calyx, and with a very large 3-lobed lower lip, borne in axillary whorls, sometimes forming a short terminal cluster. Stems long slender 30-60 cm., prostrate, creeping and rooting at the nodes; leaves long-stalked, with rounded or oblong, shalowly lobed blade with a heart-shaped base, 2.5-4 cm.

Flowering and fruiting: April-May

Distribution: Central Nepal to South-West China, Burma. 1500-3000 meter alt. Forests, shrubberies.

Ajuga parviflora Benth.

Softly villous herb. Stems spreading delicately branched from the base. Leaves shorly stalked or sessile, ovate or oblong, 5-15 cm. long, toothed or almost entire, lower surface often tinged with pupple; radical leaves spreading. Flowers small about 6 mm., blue crowded in axilllary, whorls forming leafy spikes, floral leaves smaller. Corolla-tube straight, hardly longer than the calyx, blue stamens 4, in marginal pairs, included within the tube. Nutlets very small, rugosely pitted.

Flowering and fruiting:	March-Octobe:
Distribution:	Western Himalaya, Temperate regions from Kashmir to Kumaon 2000-2300m.; Siwaliks. Afghanistan.

Ajuga species found in Siwaliks, the plains, and hilly region may be distinguished by their floral characterstics. Flowers pale or liliac and stamens protruding in *Ajuga remota* Benth., whereas flowers are blue and the stamens included in *Ajuga parviflora* Benth. In general various spécies of genus *Ajuga* may differ in characters of flowers. Calyx-lobes acute, corolla-tube erect and not inuced at base in *Ajuga bracteosa,* when *Ajuga macrosperama* has obtuse or rounded calyx-tube and inflated corolla-tube at base and geniculate above the swollen base. Morphologically, the habit salient features may broadly separate these species. Plants with ascending stems only are of *Ajuga bracteosa* and *A. lupulina,* whereas the plant with creeping stems rooting at the nodes are of *Ajuga lobata.*

Genus *Ajuga* in family Lamiaceae or Labiatae, with salient features - Softly hairy herbs; stems erect or ascending. Leaves ovate or oblong. Flowers small, crowded in axillary whorls forming leafy spikes, more or less interrupted near the base. Calyx ovoid; teeth 5, acute, nearly equal. Corolla tube slightly dilated at the mouth; limb 2-lipped, upper lip very short erect, flat, 2-lobed, lower much longer, spreading, 3-lobed, lateral equal pairs, protruding from under the upper lip or included in the tube.

30 species of the temperate Old World.

Genus *Ajuga* Linn. with about 100 palaeotemperate species, and seven species in India, confined in the Himalayas and the hills of Chota Nagpur, and other regions, belongs to tribe 7 Ajugoideae having common features-calyx 10-nerved, stamens 4, ascending, ovary 4-lobed, nutlets smooth, thick or fleshy, with a small basal areola. Genus *Ajuga* with specific characters upper corolla lip short notched, usually shorter than the incurved stamens; and distinguishes from other genera *Leucosceptrum* Smith., *Teucrium* Linn. and *Cymaria* Benth. in the group.

There are about 8 species in the Himalayan region of genus *Ajuga* Bugle-corolla with a very short upper lip and a large 3-lobed lower lip, and corolla-tube with a ring of hairs within, calyx with 5 nearly equal lobes; and *Ajuga* and other some genera *Teucrium, Mentha, Elsholtzia* and *Leucosceptrum* have corolla with 4-5 nearly equal lobes, or with upper lip absent or very short which are distinguishing characters of flower from other genera.

The root, root bark, leaves and whole plant of *Ajuga bracteosa* Wall. ex Benth. are medicinally useful.

Whole plant is bitter, astringent, aromatic, tonic and useful in agues. Leaves are useful in fever and also considered a substitute for cinchona.

The plant yields ceryl alcohol, B-sitosterol, Y-sitosterol, cerotic and palmitic acids and a glucosidic coanstituent.

The aromatic leaves are considered as stimulant, diuretic and aperient.

Root bark is useful as anthelmintic in worms complaints, and also useful as purgative in constipation and other abdominal troubles. Whole plant is useful in fever, cold, coryza, periodic fevers, malaria, gonorrhoea and other ailments. Leaves are useful in syphilis. Leaves are useful as blood purifier and in ailments caused with impurity of blood. Leaves are useful in burns, boils and erruptions.

Whole plant of *Ajuga macrosperma* Benth. are edible as vegetable.

The plant drug Jan-in-adam is regarded as a bitter astringent, nearly inodorous, sometimes substituted for cinchona in the treatment of fevers by preparing infusion or in other forms. Mukand-babri is used (in Salt Range) to kill lice, and is regarded as depurative. It is an aromatic tonic useful in general debility and other similar conditions.

Ajuga chamaeptys Schraber syn. *Teucrium chamaepitys* is plant source for Unani drug, Khamaphinus known in Arabic or Persian medical compendium. Similarly, the plant *Teucrium chaeaedrys* Linn. (Wall Germander) is source for Unani drug Khamaidrus incorporated there.

Medicinal properties and action of plant drug *Ajuga bracteosa* Wall ex Benth.-Rasa Tikta-katu-kaṣāya Vipāka Kaṭu, Virya Usna, Vatakapha nasaka. Pittasāṁsam ana (Tridosahara); and Karma Balya, Jvaraghna, Dahaprasamana, Kṛmighna, Sāraka, Mūtrala, Grāhī, Uttejaka, Raktaprasādana, Tvacya, Ropaṇa, and thereapeutic uses as internal and external application in Jvar Jvara,, Āmavata, Vatarakta, Pratisyāya, Visaṁajvara, Upadamsa, Phiraṅga Vṛṇa, Agnidagdha, Visphoṭa, Vibandha, Mutrāghata, Udaravikāra, Dāha, Raktaduṣṭi, Tvacāvikāra and other diseases.

Nīlakaṇṭhī, the Sanskrit name for plant drug *Ajuga bracteosa* Wall. ex Benth:

4

Anisomeles indica (Linn.) Kuntze.

Nepeta indica Linn.

Anisomeles ovata R.Br.

A. ovata Aiton.

Epimeredi indicus (Linn.) Rothm.

Family: Lamiaceae (Labiatae)

Regional names: Parpata, Kala bhangr, Kala cheeta, Ramtulsi, Basinga, Narutami, Perunkurinja; Gopuli (Bombay);

Suffruticose herb, 3-4 ft. high, sparingly hairy to densely pubescent or almost woolly. Stems acutely 4-angled. Leaves 2.5-3 in. long, ovate, acute, crenate-serrate, thickly herbaceous, softly pubescent on both sides, base truncate rounded or rarely cuneate, the margins entire; petiole densely hairy. Whorls axillary, many flowered, more or less interrupted below, crowded above, the whorl forming a dense spicate inflorescence; bracts 1.5-1.8 in. long, linear, clothed with long stiff-hairs. Calyx subsessile, enlarging in fruit hirsute; calyx teeth about as long as the tube, lanceolate acute, ciliate. Corolla 5/8 in. long; upper lip pale-purple 1/4 in. long, oblong, rounded-lower tip deep blue, much longer the midlobe deeply 2-fid. Filaments bearded. Nutlets 1/10 in. long, smooth shining and black when ripe.

Flowering and fruiting: Flowers paste-rainy season; January-December; June-October; September-March

Distribution: Throughout India and in Ceylon ascending to 5,000 ft. alt. in the

Himalayas, extending to the Malay Peninsula and Islands to China and the Philippines.

Anisomeles indica (Linn.) O. Kuntze.

Erect, aromatic, annual-perennial herbs. Stems acutely 4-angular, densely short-hairy. Leaves ovate-lanceolate to oblong, with a rounded-cordate to cuneate base, acute or acuminate crenate-serrate, thinly hairy to densely pubescent, 3-15 x 1-5-8 cm. Petioles 1.5-8 cm. long. Verticillasters few to many-flowered, combined into spikes. Bracts linear-spatulate, 0.4-1 cm. long. Calyx 0.8-1 cm. long, hairy, gland-dotted; teeth 0.22-0.3 cm. long. Corolla bluish purple, 1.5-2 cm. long. Nutlets ovoid, polished 0.15-0.17 cm. long.

Genus *Anisomeles* R. Br. in family Lamiaceae or Labiatae, has about 7 species in Indo-Malesia and Australia; and herbs, 3 species in Southern India, with 1 extending to the Himalayas (1,650 m.).

Anisomeles indica (Linn.) O. Kuntze. is very variable in habit, size and shape of leaves, degree of haiiness and number of flowers in a verticillasters.

A form of this plant, *Aiisomeles mollissima* Wall., with densely woolly pubescent and regarded as deserving varietal rank which is aboundant in Siwaliks and Upper Gangetic plains with this plant species.

Genus *Epimeredi* Adanson is sometimes considered as cogeneric with *Anisomeles* R. Brown.

Genus *Anisomeles* R. Br. with salient features-Foliar bracts large in pairs, linear. Calyx tubular, 10-nerved, equally 5-lobed. Corolla 2-lipped; tube annulate within; upper lip entire, flat; lower lip larger, with 4-spreading lobes. Stamens 4, `didynamous; filaments beraded, anterior pair the longest and exerted; anthers dimorphic; lower 2, each with 2 transverse paralled cells; upper 2 dimidiate (1-celled).

Two species of the genus *Anisomeles* R. Br. differ on the basis of distinguishing characterstics: Leaves ovate and under-shrubs are greyish tomentose of *Anisoemels indica* (L.) Kuntze.; whereas leaves lanceolate in white tomentose undershrubs of *Anisomeles malabarica* (L.) R. Br.

Various genera in family Labiatae (64 genera with 380 species in India chiefly in mountainous regions) are broadly distinguished on the basis of flower and leaves characterstics. In view of genus *Anisomeles* R. Br., various the genera are with ovary 4-partite, areola of nutlets small and balilar or placed somewhat obliquely to the outer side; stamens 4, all perfect and declinate, anther-cells at length confluent; and attachment of nutlets basllar; and lower lip of corolla declinate, flat or slightly concave, generally narrower but hardly longer than the 3-4-lobed upper lip. Among such genera, the genus *Anisomeles* R. Br. has specific characters in flowers: Upperlip of corolla short, nearly flat; anthers of upper stamens 2-celled, of lower 1-celled, the cells transverse add parallel and the genus belong to the genera having erect spreading or ascending stamens 4 all perfect; and calyx 5-10 nerved, corolla 2-lipped, stamens didynamous and anterior or stamens the longer.

Plant quite commonly occurring in the areas of Upper Gangetic Plains, Siwaliks and adjoining areas; frequently in waste places, roadsides, forest clearings and scrub jungles.

Anisomeles indica (Linn.) Kuntze. An erect, woody herb to undershrub, 1-2 m. high. high, branching from the base. Stems shortly 4-winged, woolly-hairy. Leaves 5-10x3.5-7 cm., ovate, cordate, crenate-serrate, scaberulous. Flowers 2x6 cm., dark red, in many-flowered, axillary whorls forming a dense, interrupted, spicate inflorescence. Calyx accrescent. Nutlets black, smooth, polished.

Plant common on moist soils of fruit gardens as a shrubby undergrowth or along the slopes of canal banks and many other places. Delhi, Haryana and Punjab, various parts of northern India, Uttar Pradesh, Bihar.

Anisomeles indica (L.) Kuntze. Undershrubs with stems acutely tetrgonous, greyish tomentose. Blade ovate, truncate-cordate, upto 5x3 cm. Cymes sessile, sometimes shrotly peduncled in fruit. Corolla bluish-white to pink.

Indomalaysia, China. Occasional across the plains; in partial or full sun on dry, soil; Karnataka; southern India; Central India, Madhya Pradesh; Western India, Gujarat, Maharastra.

Anisomeles malabarica (L.) R. Br.

Nepeta malabarica L.
Anisomeles disticha
Epimeredi malabarica (L.) Rothm.
Anisomeles fruticosa
Family: Llamiaceae (Labiatae)
Regional names: Chodhara (Marathi), Moga-biraku, Maga-bisa (Telgu), Priya-meruti, Peyameratti (Tamil), Karitumbe (Kannarese), Karithumba (Malayalam), Mogbeeraku (Telgu), Kalothumbo (Konkan), Malabar Catmint (English), Magbir-kapatta; Bulan-sachun (Santals).

Shrubby plant, 4-6 ft. high, with aromatic leaves, silvery tomentose undershrubs; stem obtusely tetragonous. Leaves lanceolate, round at base, upto 9 x 2.5 cm.; stem obtusely tetragonus. Calyx accrescent. Corolla pink.

Plant occurring in south India and Ceylon.

Mauritius, Indomalaysia. Karnataka, Malabar Coast, Travance. The whole plant of *Anisomeles indica* (L.) Kuntze.

has a strong scent resembling camphor. It is characterstic aromatic herb growing in many parts frequently in country.

The plant *Anisomeles malabarica* R. Br. yields an essential oil (roots and stems 0.006%, leaves 0.025% and flowers 0.07%) containing citral. Triperpenic acid is isolated which is identified as betulinic acid.

Pharmacognostic characters of the roots and leaves of *Anisomeles malabrica* R. Br. are in macro and micro features.

Leaves are simple, thick, velvette, petiolate, lanceolate, to oblong, acute, rounded at the base with bluntly serrate margins. Leaf is pubescent in both surfaces.

Leaf is dorsiventral. Prsesence of small cubical epidermal cells both on petiole as well as in midrib, long multi-seriate, uniseriate glandular hairs with 3-4 basal cells. sessile glandular hairs in the lamina; diacytic stomata on both the surfaces and acicular calcium oxalate crystals in the ground tissue of petiole and midrib.

Tap roots have dirty yellowish surface and whitish wood. The fracture is fibrous. The external surface has numerous longitudinal wrinkles and scars of rootlets.

Diagnostic features of the roots are the presence of elliptical to oval shaped stone cells in phelloderm, funnel shaped medullary rays in the phloem region, relatively scanty percentage of vessels and abundant tracheids and simple starch grains in the ray cells.

Anisomeles heyneana Br.

Anisomeles heyneana Benth.

Tecucrium secundum Heyne.

Family: Lamiaceae (Labiatae)

Regional names: Phagulu

Erect corase herb. Sparsely hairy of glabrate leaves, ovate-lanceolate, acuminate, cuneate-serrate, leaves 2-3 in. green, petioles about 1/8-1/2 in. Cymes peduncled lax-fid, sometimes elongate and many-flowered; bracts small, subulate. Calyx hispid, teeth triangular-lanceolate acuminate, margins fringed. Corolla white, broadly oblong, polished.

Distribution: Deccan Peninsula; Western Ghats, from the Concan Southwards.

Perhaps it is only a variety of *Anisomeles ovata* R. Br. The leaves of the plant and also whole herb are medicinally useful. Leaves are considered useful against headache.

Anisomeles indica (Linn.) Kuntze. is useful as astringent and carmiative. Whole plant is considered tonic. Oil from plant is useful in uterine affections.

The leaves, roots, oil and whole plant of *Anisomeles indica* (L.) Ktz. are medicinally useful.

Whole plant is useful as antipyretic, anodyne, astringent, carminative, refrigerant nervine tonic; and used in fevers, dyspepsia, stomach troubles, bowel complaits, diarrhoea, muscular pains, heat sensation and nervine debility. Roots are useful is antidote to poisonous bites. Leaves are useful in swelling of neck and wounds.

In veterinary medicine, the whole plant is considered useful in dysentery and bowel troubles of animals.

This plant is known as Chodhara in Maharastra or particularly Bombay which is meant for four-angled, and it is good aromatic plant. There was previous (during 1980 reports that it was included among the plants which are sold in Bombay market as gao-suban (but it is not gule-gao-suban). Probably it was known by this name in kutch, but true gao-suban (*Echium)* was imported from Persia that time.

The leaves, oil and whole plant of *Anisomeles malabarica* R.Br. are medicinally useful.

Leaves are useful as stomachic, carminative, diaphoretic and astringent. Essential oil is used externally in rheumatism. The plant is useful in scorpion-sting and snake-bite.

Essential oil distilled from leaves or decoction of whole plant is employed externally in rheumatism.

Infusion of leaves is used in colic and dyspepsia, catarrhal affections, and intermittent fevers, and given to children suffering with colic, abdominal troubles, dyspepsia and teething troubles specially fever, diarrhoea and gripes or bowel complaints.

Infusion of aromatic bitter leaves is considered quite common recipe in affections of the stomach and bowels, catarrhal affections and intermittent fevers. Besides the oral use for drinking as liquid form, the patients are also made to inhale the vapour of a hot infusion so as to induce copious diaphoresis. Similar application of vapour is useful in coryza, cold and other catarrhal affections. Vapour bath of leaves is also useful for profuse diaphoresis.

Medicinal properties and action of plant drug-Rasa tikta-kaṣāya, Vīrya uṣṇa, Vipāka kaṭu, Guṇa anuśnasita laghnu, Vatapiṭṭahara (tridoṣāsamaka); and Karma stambhana, grahi, jvaraghana, vedanāsthāpana, dīpana, pācana, svedajanana, sothahara, vātānulomana, balya, viṣaghna, vraṇaropaṇa, sitala, sugandhita, nāḍībalya, and pratisyāyahara.

Therapeutic indication in Jvara, kasa, pratisyāya, bālaroga-dantodbheda vikāra-udarasūla-vikāra, āmavāta, dāha, tṛṣṇā, sotha, vraṇa, vṛnasotha, atisāra, āmāsayavikāra, udaravikāra, pravāhikā, sula, vātavyādhi, nāḍīdaurbalya, kāsa, udarasūla and other various ailments.

Pasucikitsā-Udararoga, atisāra land sūla.

Vaikuṇṭha, Bhūtānkusha and Gandhapatrā, the Sanskrit names for plant drug.

5

Apama siliquosa Lamk.

Bragantia wallichii R.Br. ex. W. & A.

Family: Aristolochaaceae

Regional names: Chakrani (Marathi), Niruvale (Kannarese), Alpam (Malayalam), Tellayeshwari (Telgu); Kuravan-kanda

Erect shrub or subscandent undershrub. Leaves subsessile, up to 22 x 6 cm., elliptic-lanceolate, acute, narrowed at base, sparsely hairy. Perianth lobes ovate-orbicular, acute, fleshy, externally hairy, dark purple. Stamens 6, in 3 groups of 2, adnate in style; anthers hairy. Fruit elongate, narrowly cylindrical; seeds 3-gonous, pitted.

Distribution: Western Peninsular India, Sri lanka. Common, in shade of forests under growth amidst boulders or on banks or forests streams; Karnataka.

Flowering and fruiting: February-March

Bragantia wallichii R.Br. syn. *Apama siliquosa* Lam.

An erect shrub of the Deccan Peninsula and Ceylon; it is common in the evergreen forests around Gerosppa falls and in South Konkan.

Bragantea Linn. is a genus of 5 species of shrubs and under shrubs, distributed in India and Malaya; 4 of these are found in India.

Bragantia tomentosa Blume syn. *Apama tomentosa* Engl. are *Bragantia wallichii* R.Br. are medicinal.

Genus *Apama* Lamarack. syn. Bragantia Linn. with salient fetures-Erect, subscandent undershrubs. Leaves usually triplenerved. Inflorescence of axillary cymes of short racemes. Flowers actinomorphic. Perianth lobes spreading. Stamens 6-12, free or in groups of 2 and adnate to style, connective, slightly produced. Ovary 4-locular, style 4-fid. Capsule 4-valved; seeds not winged.

Genus *Apama* Lamk. has specific characters in the family Aristolochiaceae. Erect undershrub, perianth tubular below and free above are major features of *Apama* Lamk.; whereas the genus *Aristolichia* Linnaeus has herbaceous twiners, with perianth inflated and ventricose in lower half, obliquely elongate above.

The roots leaves and whole plant of *Bragantic wallichii* R.Br. syn. *Apama siliquosa* Linn. are medicinally useful.

The roots are useful in cholera, diarrhoea and dysenthery. Whole plant is mixed with oil and made into an ointment considered to be benefecial for carbuncles and inverterate ulcers.

The mature roots are used in treatment of dysentery. They are ground to a paste with lemon juice (60 gr. in 1/2 oz.) and administered orally every 15 minutes.

Plant considered useful as sedative.

The pharmacological studies record the observations. The plant was tested for vibriocidal as well as anti-cholera activity. None of the extracts had any vibriocidal activity, although the pure base was active in vitro against S. typhi and E. coli. However, the pure base was found to prevent death of rabbits suffering from cholera when given in an early stage (i.e. one hour before infection). The drug had no benefecial effect after onset of diarrhoea.

The phytochemical screening finds that the roots contain isoristolochic acid, $C_{17}H_{11}O_7N$, which was first isolated from *Aristolochia indica.* Qualitative tests indicated the presence of alkaloids, but no pure base could be isolated.

The roots are considered useful in stomachache, chest pain, headache, indigestion, skin diseases and dysentery and similar bowel complaints.

The ointment prepared with roots in oil said to very efficacious in the treatment of psora or inveterate ulcers. Like other plants belonging to the same family, it is supposed to have virtues in the cure of snake bites.

Plant is useful as an antidote to snake-bite. The leaves juice mixed with the roots of Vacā *(Acorus calamus)*, the root itself rubbed up with lime-juice, and made into a poultice and externally applied, are the chief modes of administering it among the natives. This is regarded of as one of the most powerful antidotes to poison known on the west coast.

About the efficacy of plant against snake-bite or as antidote to poison, a Malabar proverb says "As soon as the Alpam root enters the body, the poison leaves it."

Apama tomentosa (Bl.) Engl.

Ceramium tomentosum Bl.

Bragantia tomentosa Bl.

The roots, leaves and whole plant of *Apama tomentosa* (Bl.) Engl. are medicinally useful.

The plant is bitter and is regarded as an emmenagogue. Leaves are used in cough; and given as diuretic. Whole plant is considered useful in skin diseases, snake bite, scorpion and insect stings and boils.

The plant is also a fish poison.

Another species of the genus *Bragantia* Linn. found in India is *Apama dalzellii* (Hook.f.) Kuntze. syn. *Bragantia dalzellii* Hoo.f.

The roots of *Bragantia wallichii* R.Br. contain alkaloid chakranine.

The wood of the stem of *Bragantia* Linn. is very peculiar, differing in a remarkable degree from that of the ordinary exogens.

The pharmacognostic characters of the plant *Apama siliquosa* Linn. find that the roots of plants were observed to grow very long in comparison to stem and is tortuous, profusely branched, greyish cream with an oily odour add a bitter taste. Deep longitudinal fissures appear on the surface of the root resụlting in the formation of prominent elongated islands, pointed at both the ends, lenticels being quite large. The root bark is transection has 4-10 layers of rectangular to squarish thick walled cells with a dark brown deposit. Stellar cylinder is very prominent, medullary rays are very broad and have hexagonal cells. The powder of the root is yellowish green. Bark cells are impregnated with tannin and cork cells with subrin. Starch is present in the cells of pericycle. Medullary ray cells have abundance of starch and sugars. Some of the cells are sclerosed.

Medicinal properties and action of plant drug-Rasa tikta-kaṣāya, Vīrya uṣṇa, Vipāka kaṭu, Guna laghu, Tridoṣahara (vātapittāsamaka); and Karma viṣaghna, grāhi, sāmaka, vedanāsthāpana, vraṇaropaṇa, Jīvāṇuhara, javraghna, tvacya, kāsaghna, mūtrala, ārtavajanana dīpana and pācana.

Therapeutic indication in Atisāra, pravāhikā viṣūcikā, jvara, tvagvikāra, vraṇa, pramehapiḍikā, diṣṭavraṇa, kāsa, sarpadaṁsa, kītadaṁsa, yāngamaviṣa, ārtavavikāra-rajorodha, udaravikara, agnimandya, sirasūla, urahsūla, ajīrṇa, mūtravikāra and other various ailments.

Cakraṇī, the Sanskrit name for plant drug.

6

Borreria articularis (L.f.) F.N. Williams

Spermacoce hispida L.

Spermacoce articularis L.f.

Borreria hispida (L.) K. Schum.

Spermacoce scabra Willd.

Family: Rubiaceae

Regional names: Ghantachibaji, Dhati (Bombay), Piluna-arak (Santals), Nattaichuri, (Tamil), grendhi, Madana, Madina, Madan-budat-kada, Madana (Telgu,) Madanaghanti (Hindi); Kairkar, kurgimandor, Solaganthi, Burdmutta, Satgathiya, Ghathiyaghas, Gatbhanyan.

Procumbent herb with hispid hairy of sub-glabrous stems. Leaves subsessile, 1/2-1.5 in. long, obovate, spathulate oblong or elliptic, acute or obtuse, rigidly coriaceous, pale when dry, usually very scabrid above; margins often thickened and cartilaginous, sacbrid or ciliate; stipules membranous, hispid, bristly. Flowers 4-6 in. a whorl, shortly pedicelled; bracteoles aw long as the calyx; filiform, hyaline. Calyx 1/2 in. long, hispid; teeth linear-lanceolate, acute, reflexed, equalling the tube. Corolla 1/4-1/2 in., blue; lobes oblong, acute, bristly outside. Stamens 2, very short. Capsules 1/2 in. long, pubescent or hispid, rounded at the base, crowned with the the calyx-teeth, one carpel dehiscing ventrally. Seeds not polished.

Flowering and fruiting: June-December; August-October; March-November

Distribution: Subtropical Himalayas from the neighbourhood of Shimla eastwards, and south to Ceylon; also in the Malay Peninsula and Islands, China and Phillippines.

Plant occurring as a very abundant weed within the areas of Upper Gangetic Plains, Siwaliks and adjacent regions.

Borreria articularis (L.f.) F.N. William syn. *B. hispida* L.

Initially erect, then procumbent, hispid herbs. Leaves elliptic-lanceolate, up to 3 x 1 cm. Calyx 4-lobed. Corolla bluish-blue. Mericarps pubescent, with septum on emericarp, septum finally separating.

Indomalyasia. Fairly common across the plain and in Upper Ghats, Karnataka; Southern India.

Borreria hispida K. Schum.

A procumbent, deep-rooted annual. Branches quadrangular. Leaves decussate, ovate, ovate-oblong or elliptic-oblong, 3-4 x 1.5-2 cm., leathery. Flowers pale blue or pale violet, in nodal whorls, tetramerous, erect. Capsules about 4x2 mm., oblong, hairy, both carpels dehiscing ventrally. Seeds oval, dark brown, grooved ventrally.

Plant occurring in Delhi area and adjoining region; plant comes on the Ridge during the monsoon period, and also found in the plains as a weed in cultivated and unused grounds on damp, sandy soils.

Borreria articularis (Linn. f.) F.N. Williams syn. *Spermacoce hispida* Linn. (non *Borreria hispida* Spruce ex K. Schum)

Erect or decumbent-ascending, annual-perennial herbs, with a stout tap roots. Stems 4-angular, often many from the woody base, hispidly hairy on the angles. Leaves lanceolate-oblong or obovate, acute, often narrowed into a short petiole towards the base, acute at apex, sacbrid along undulate margins, glabrous or thinly strigose, 0.5-2.5 (-3) X 0.4-1.5 cm. long. Flowers in clusters at the ends of much reduced, axillary branchlets. Calyx-lobes subequal, lanceolate, 0.2-0.25 cm. long. Corolla whitish or pale-purple, with a ring of hairs just above the base of the tube; lobes lanceolate, obtuse, 0.2 cm. long, hairy outside. Style 0.5-0.6 cm. long, short-hairy. Fruit obvoid, hispdly hairy at the top, 0.4 x 0.25 cm., septum detached from the valves when spreading. Seeds 0.25 X 1.0-0.12 cm.

Plant common in sandy, grassy localities, fields, roadsides, sal forests and waste places; Siwaliks, northern India.

Genus *Borreria* G.F.W.Mey in the family Rubiaceae Juss., has about 150 species in warmer regions of the world; annual or perennial herbs, 7 species in India; 2 species occur throughout India, and the rest confined to Western and Southern India, ascending up to 1,650 m. in the Himalayas.

A genus consisting of nearly 100 species mainly of annual and perennials herbs, distributed in tropical countries. It is represented in India by 3 or 4 species. Several species of genus *Borreria* Mey are medicinal.

Borreria pusilla (Wall.) DC.

Borreria brachystema (R. Br. ex Benth.) Valet.

Spermacoce brachystema R. Br. ex Benth.

S. stricta Linn. f. (non *B. stricta* G.F.W. Meyer)

Borreria stricta (Linn. f.) K.Schum.

Spermacoce pusilla Wall.

Family: Rubiaceae

Erect, simple or rarely branched only at the top, annual herbs. Stems scabrid on angles. Leaves linear-lanceolate to oblong, acute at apex, glabrous or scabrid, whitish on the lower surface, 2-6 X 0.3-1 cm. Stipule-bristles 4-5, 0.5-0.6 cm.

long. Flowers in dense, terminal clusters, rarely in axillary clusters. Bracts of flowers filiform, 0.3-0.3.35 cm. long. Calyx-lobes linear-lanceolate, acute, mucronate, 0.12-0.15 cm. long. Stamens 3-4, exerted. Corolla white or pale-purple, 0.3 cm. long, lobes ovate, obtuse, 0.1-0.12 cm. long. Fruit obvoid, hispidly hairy at the top, 0.3 cm. long, with completely disappearing septum. Seeds 0.25 X 0.1-12 cm., flocculate.

Floering and fruiting:	March-November; October-December; All seasons.
Distribution:	Tropical Himalayas from Kashmir eastwards up to 5,500 ft. elevation; and throughout India to Ceylon, Burma, the Malay Peninsula and China.

Spermacpce stricta Linne. f. sy. *Borreria stricta* Linn. f. Annual herbs. Stems erect, 6-14 in. high; simple or branched from the base, angles more or less scabrid with recurved prickles. Leaves sub-sessile, spreading or ultimately reflexed, 1-2 in long, linear to ovate, acute and often mucronate, more or less coriaceous, glabrous or scabrid, margins often recurved stipules with many long bristles. Flowers many, in globose compact axillary heads; bracteoles filifrom exceeding the calyx. Calyx-tube pubescent above, glabrous near the base; calyx-teeth linear-subulate. Corolla white, tube very slender; lobes linear, acute. Stigma sub-globose. Capsule narrowed at the base, glabrous below, rather membranous crowned with the erect calyx-teeth, both carpels dehiscing ventrally. Seeds polished.

Plant occurring in the Upper Gangetic Plains; Bundelkhand, Rohilkhand, Uttar Pradesh; northern India, central India and other various parts of country.

Borreria stricta (Linn. f.) K. Schum. An erect, small herb. stems short, scabrid with recurved, scabrous hairs. Leaves whorled, ovate-oblong or linear. Stipules united into a tube, filiform-bristly. Flowers many, in dense, axillary and terminal culsters.

Plant occurs rarely on the Ridge amongst the cervices of rocks and on reddish-brown sandstones, Delhi; and adjacent areas in the regions.

Borreria pusilla (Wall.) DC. syn. *B. stricta* Linn. f.

Erect herbs. Leaves ovate-lanceolate, up to 4X0.6 cm. Calyx 4-lobed. Corolla white. Mericarps pubescent, separating from septum.

Plant distributed in Paleotropics. Scattered across plains. Karnataka; Southern India.

Genus *Borreria* G.F. Meyer, formerly included under the genus *Spermacoce* Linn., is recognizable by companulate-urceolate, white, rarely light purple-tinged corolla, 2 or 4-8 calyx-lobes, stamens being in serted on the throat of corolla and capsule-septum being either detached from valves ornot, if not detached., then it splits longitudinally; whereas the genus *Spermacoce* Linn. is characterized by infundibuliform, purple corolls, 4 calyx-lobes, stamens being inserted near the base of corolla-tube and caosule being persistently attached to one valve, with the other valve being detached from the septum and opened on the ventral side.

In the family Rubiaceae (about 500 genera with over 6,000 species, and about 76 genera with 274 in India), many genera are grouped majorly on the basis of fruit-characters (particularly genera in northern India and other regions); and the genus *Borreria* Mey belongs to genera bearing 2-seeded fruits, and with specific characters such as Inflorescences axillary or terminal, of clusters of flowers, and fruit dehiscent into 2-dehiscent cocci. Stipules present, leaves opposite, plants otherwise (herbs), flowers not in capitate heads and other characters of flower and its organs.

Among the erect or prostrate herbs of family particularly certain genera, the genus Borreria Meyer has flowers whorled or in axillary heads; whereas genus *Oldenlandia* Linn. flowers in axillalry and terminal, and cymes paniculate. Genus *Spermacoce* Linn. belongs to tribe XV Spermacoceae of Indian genera of Rubiaceae family, comprising three genera *Hydrophylax* Linn., *Spermacoce* Linn. and *Gallonia* A. Rich; and the genus *Spermacoce* is specific for fruit of 2 separable cocci and both or one only dehiscing ventrally.

Mainly the species of Indian subcontinent carry various of differences as well as similarity.

Two important species of *Borreria* G.F.W. Meyer initially differ on the basis of habit and flower colour. *Borreria stricta* (Linn. f.) K.Schum is of erect small herbs bearing white flowers, when the herbs larger and procumbent having pale blue or pale violet flowers in *Borreria hispida* K. Schum. Former species or sometimes often escapes notice by its small size, or it is distinguishable due to smaller herb primarily. Latter is very variable in habit, hairiness and size and shape of leaves. This may be represented by cytotypes and (or) ecotypes in different habitats.

These species differ by their flower characters. *Borreria brachystema* (R.Br. ex Benth) Valet. syn. *B. stricta* (Linn.) K. Schum annuals are of flower-clusters many-flowered, with exerted flower-bracts, and their corolla 0.3 cm. long; whereas corolla 0.8-1.5 cm. long in perennials of *Borreria articularis* (Linn. f.) F.N. Williams syn. *B. hispida* (Linn.) K. Schum., with flower-clusters few-flowered, without flower-bracts.

Borreria stricta (Linn. f.) K. Schum. syn. *Spermacoce stricta* Linn. f. is distinguishable from *Borreria hispida* (L.) K. Schum. syn. *Spermacoce hispida* Linn. by their stems and carpels. Stems erect and both carpels dehiscing ventrally in *Borreria stricta;* whereas stems procumbent and one carpel dehiscing ventrally and the other remaining indehiscent in *Borreria hispida.*

Some other species of the genus *Borreria* Linn. may also be mentioned which have relevance to important species:

Borreria ocymoides (H. Burma) DC

Spermacoce ocymoides N. Burman

S. Stricta Schlect.

Erect herbs. Leaves elliptic-ovate, subacute, up to 3.5 x 1.5 cm. Calyx lobes 4, unequal. Corolla white. Mericarps each covered by septum.

Distribution in Tropics. Rare in Ghats, Karnataka; Southern India. Flowering in July-October.

Borreria repens DC.

Spermacoce ocymoides auct. non Burm. f.

B. setidens auct. non Ridley

Perennial; Western Peninsula, from Malabar and the Niligri hills southwards. Malacca, Malay Islands, Mauritius, Tropical Africa.

Borreria verticillata (L.) G.F.W. Meyer

Spermacoce verticillata L.

Large herbs or subshrubs. Leaves oblong-lanceolate, up to 5 X 1 cm. Heads subterminal. Calyx 2-lobed. Corolla white. Mericarps pubescent, each covered by septum.

Distribution in Pantropics. Plant introduced and naturalised, fairly common in open grounds across the plain, Karnataka; Southern India. Flowering in all season.

Spermacoce ascaberrima Blume.

Herb rather stout, 12-16 in. Leaves brown when dry; branches ascending rather shining, nearly glabrous but scabrid or hairy. Leaves elliptic or elliptic-lanceolate, acute scabrid above with deeply impressed nerves. Capsule glabrous; seeds oblong granulate shining.

Distribution in Sumtra, Java, Burma, Malacca.

A few other species of *Borreris* Meyer may be indicated in addition to foregoing species;-

Borreria alata (Aubl.) DC

Spermacoce alata Aubl.

S. latifolia Aubl.

Borreria latifolia (Aubl.) K. Schum.

B. cradii Ravi.

Borreria repens DC.

Spermacoce ocymoides acut. non Burm. f.

Borreria setidens auct. non Ridley

Borreria rosea (S. & M.) Sivarajan.

B. stricta (L. f.) K. Schum. var. *rosea* S. & M.

The roots, seeds and whole plant of *Borreria hispida* (Linn.) K. Schum are medicinally useful.

The decoction of the roots is used as alterative. Seeds are useful as stimulant. The vapour of plant boiled into water is inhaled to kill tooth worms and considered useful in dental carries.

The seeds are employed to prepare infusion and said to be used as coffee drink, and also its substitute.

The leaves are eaten in time of scarcity. They are also used as a vegetable which is also some times used in scarcity, or as vegetables in general.

The plant is used as fodder for cattles.

The roots, which are little thicker than the official Sarsaparilla root, like that, used as an alterative. It may be given in decoction to the extent of 4 ounces or more daily suiting to patients and ailments.

The roots are useful as antidote to snake bite They are employed to prepare decoction and given after short intervals in beginning stage.

As an antifertility drug, the roots are considered useful. The roots infusion or decoction is given to women desiring contraception.

In some female diseases, the plant is useful. The decoction or infusion of the roots is given to ladies in cases of excess bleeding in child birth. In the stage of miscarriage and premature bleeding during pregnancy and in the abortion, the roots are considered useful as oral medicine for checking the ailing conditions.

The roots infusion of plant is given in loss of appetite as appetiser or stimulating the appetite. It is useful in conditions of appetite loss or also as stomachic.

Whole plant in decotion form, also as powder, is orally considered useful in bodyache and also as nervine tonic or stimulant in general.

The roots are useful in toothache, gum troubles, life complaints, ulcers, swellings and wounds. They are applied externally in the ailments and also in other similar forms. The leaves are particularly useful in ulcers, wounds, scabies, skin diseases and eruptions.

Medicinal properties and action of the plant drug-Rasa tikta-kasaya, Vīrya uṣṇa, Vipāka kaṭu, Guṇa uṣṇa, Vātakapha nāsaka (pitta saṁsamana- tridoṣasāmaka); Karma balya, uttejaka, dīpana, kṣudhāvardhaka, tvacya, raktarodhaka, raktaprasādana, garbhasthāpana, ārtavaniyamana, vedanāsthāpana, dantya, cakṣuṣya, vraṇaropaṇa, santati niyamana, visaghna, hrdya and sothahara.

Therapeutic indication in Tvagvikāra, vraṇa, sotha, visa, sarpadaṁsa, aruci, kṣudhānāsa, atyārtava, garbhasrīva, dantaroga-dantamulasotha, dantasula and kṛmidanta, angamarda, nāḍībalya, netraroga and other āmayaka-prayoga in various diseases. It is also a patra Sāka dravya.

Madanaghaṇṭī, the Sanskrit name for plant drug.

7

Commelina benghalensis Linn.

Family: Commelinaceae

Regional names: Kanteri, Kanvo, Kankavwa, Kankaua, Kannateva, Kana (Hindi); Kanavachai (Tamil), Vennadavkura (Telgu), Kannaguharvi (Tamil); Buchna, Jeha-bhoi, Kanchara, Kanna-Manna.

Decumbent-ascending, annual herbs, with fibrous roots. Stems branched from the base, often creeping and rooting below, striate, glabrous or hairy. Leaves subsessile or narrowed into 0.4-1.5 cm. long petioles, ovate-elliptic or oblong-lanceolate, with a rounded or acute base, sub-obtuse or subacute, slightly oblique at base, glabrescent, or pubescent, ciliate, 2-10x1.5-4 cm. Sheaths pubescent, with an oblique mouth, long-ciliate, 1-1.5 cm. long. Spathes 2-3 together at the ends of branches, subsessile, cucllate, recurved, mucrinate, auricled on one side at base, hairy on the outside. Cymes on 1.5 cm. long peduncles, with 1-flowered lower branch and 2 to 3-flowered upper one. Pedicels 0.3-0.32 x 0.15 cm., lateral ones sub-orbicular-rounded, patent, 0.32x0.32 cm. Petals blue; dorsal one long-clawed, shallowly notched, 0.65-0.7 cm. long; lateral ones subsessile, 0.4 cm. long. Staminodes 3, with minute anthers. Capsule 3-gonous, short-stalked, oblong, unequally 3-valved. 0.5x0.3 cm. Seeds 5, pitted, 0.2-0.3 x 0.12-0.14 cm.

Flowering and fruiting: June or July-November; June-January.

Distribution: Throughout India, and upto 6,000 ft. alt. regions on Himalayas, extending to China and Tropical Africa.

Commelina benghalensis Linn.

Stems 2-3 ft. long, slender, dichotomously branched from the base; branches diffuse, glabrous or pubescent, creeping and rooting below. Leaves 1-3 in. long, ovate or oblong, obtuse, sessile or shrotly stalked, pubescent or villous on both surfaces; base unequal-sided, rounded cuneate or cordate, nerves 7-11 pairs; sheaths hairy, margins ciliate, with rufous hairs. Spathe 1-3 together, funnel-shaped or turbinate, auricled on the side. Sepals small, oblong, hairy. Petals blue, the larger one orbicular or transversely oblong, Ovary 3-celled, two of the cells 2-ovuled, the third cell 1-ovuled. Capsule 1/4 in. long, pyriform, membranous, 5-seeded. Seeds closely pitted.

Plant occurring in Upper Gangetic Plains and adjacent regions, Siwaliks, Bundelkhand, Rohilkhand, eastern and central India. Common on grassy localities, roadsides, waste places, waysides and fields, and many other places during rainy season.

Commelina benghalensis Linn.

A branched, diffuse or straggling herb with dimorphic flowers, creeping and rooting below. Leaves ovate to oblong, broader, obtuse, rounded, cuneate or cordate at the base. Aerial spathes 1-3 in the axils, obeonic, funnel-shaped or turbinate. Aerial flowers sky-blue to bluish-violet. Capsules 5-seeded. Seeds wrinkled, pitted. Underground flowers bisexual, usually solitary in a pear-shaped spathe.

Common rainy season annual plant occurring on the ridges and in the fields, waste places, gardens farm lands, on moist and shady places and various others localities.

Quite common in Delhi, Haryana, Punjab and other provinces in northern India, frequently in moist regions.

Commelina benghalensis L.

Subscandent herbs with underground stem naked, ending in cleistogamous, white, fertile flowers. Leaves ovate, acute, often as symmetrical at base, 2-5 x 1.5-3 cm., sheath 1 cm. long, with rufous hairs at mouth. Aerial flowers blue. Ovary 2-locular. Capsule 5-seeded.

Paleatropics; common weed in the fields of plains, Karnataka; Tamilnadu, Southern India.

This plant *Commelina benghalensis* Linn. is very variable in habit, hairiness size an shape of leaves. In this species ripe seeds are sometimes matured underground from abnormal flowers borne on leafless branches comming from the lower nodes of the stems. Those flowers are white and smaller than the blue aerial ones, which often fail to produce fertile seeds.

Commelina diffusa Burm. f.

Commelina nudiflora auct. pl. non. Linn.
Family: Commeliaceae
Regional names: Kanchura (Hindi), Vazhapazhathi (Marathi)

Diffuse, nearly glabrous herbs. Stems prostrate or subscandent, often rooting from the lower nodes. Leaves sessile, lanceolate or ovate lanceolate, acute or acuminate. Sheaths glabrous, ciliate. Spathes with a cordate or rounded base. Lateral petals obovate, long-clawed, dark blue, dorsal one, subsessile, orbicular, pale blue or white, sometimes obsolete. Capsule broadly oblong-acuminate, 5-seeded. Seeds oblong-cylindric brown tubercled and reticulate.

Plant occurring in Siwaliks and adjoining regions.

Commelina nudiflora Linn.

Commelina diffusa Burm. f.

Commelina longicaulis Jacq̄.

Commelina agraria Kunth.

Commelina salicifolia Boiger. (in past)

Commelina caespitosa Roxb.

Commelina deficiens Flor. (non. Hook. f.)

Stems creeping and rooting at the nodes or subscandent. Leaves lanceolate 1/2 by 1/3-1/3 in., glabrous scaberolous or puberlous, ciliate; spathes peduncled, ovate-lanceolate, complicate, 2/3-1 in., acute, peduncle 1/2-3/4 in., cymes 2, branches, 1-3 fid. Smaller petals blue, outer pale or white.

Distribution: Throughout the hotterparts of India, from the Punjab to Ceylon and Singapore. Tropics and Subtropics.

Murdannia nudiflora (L.) Brenan.

Commelina nudiflora L.

Aneilema nudiflorum (L.) R. Br.

Murdannia malabrics (L.) Br̂uckn.

Phaeneilema malabaricum (L.) Naray.

Trdescentia malabrica L.

Family: Commelinaceae

Diffuse slender herbs with fibrous roots. Leaves linear-lanceolate. acute or acuminate, 5x0.5 cm.; sheaths 1 cm. Panicle terminal; rachis with obscurely raised scars. Flowers purplish. Staminal filaments bearded. Capsule globose; seeds 2 per locule.

Flowering and fruiting: August-October

Pantropical. Frequent on sandy or marshy soil of plains and upper Ghats, Karnataka. Madras, Tamilnadu; Khandala, Maharastra.

Commelina longifolia Lamk.

Commelina salicifolia Roxb.

Commelina pedunculosa Link. Jahrb. (in part)
Commelina communis Wall. (in part)
Family: Commelinaceae

Regional names: Jalpipari (Hindi), Panikanchira (Bengla)

Stems slender, decumbent-ascending, rooting from the lower nodes. Leaves linear-lanceolate, glabrous. Sheaths ciliolates. Spathes axillary, ovate-lanceolate, acute or acuminate, rounded at base. Sepals ovate, obtuse; 2 lateral ones connate at base. Petals dark blue; 2 lateral ones long-clawed, ovate with undulate margins; dorsal one subsessile, ovate, entire. Seeds ovoid-subglobose, black, powdered with white, smooth, appendiculate at one end.

Commelina salicifolia Roxb.

Stem slender, diffuse, with long internodes. Leaves 3-6 by 1/4-1/2 in., nearly glabrous, sheaths ciliolate. Spathes 1/2-2 in., axillary, solitary, acute or acuminate, base rounded; branches of cymes 1-2-fid. Flowers small, dark blue. Seeds black, powdered with white.

Distribution: Java, Hong Kogg; India, from Assam and Bengal, southwards and westward to the Konkan and Coromandel.

Commelina salicifolia Roxb. Stems slender, glabrous decumbent, sometimes rooting from the nodes. Leaves 3-6 in. long, linear-lanceolate, glabrous or nearly so; sheaths 5/8 in. to 1 in., axillary ovate lanceolate, acute or acuminate, rounded at base. Peduncles 1/2-1-1/2 in. long long slender.

Flowers polygamous; branches of cyme equal, usually 1-2 fid. Sepals free, ovate, obtuse, the two inner connate below, larger than the outer. Petals dark blue, the larger ovate with undulate margins and long claws, the smaller one broadly ovate, entire, subsessile or with a very short claw. Staminodes 3, clavate. Capsule 1/4 in. long, quadrate, membranous. Seeds 1/8 in. long, black powdered with white, smooth, ovoid or subglobose, with a whithish membranous appendages at one end.

Plant occurring in the Siwalik range and Upper Gangetic Plains; Dehradun area; Sub-Himalayan tracts of north Oudh, Merwara, Rajputana, Bundelkhand.

Cummelina suffruticosa Blume.

C. semiovata Wall.

C. simsoni

C. rugulosa Clarke.

Spathodithyros suffruticous Hassk.

Family: Commelinaceae

Regional names: Darcorsa (South India)

Stems stout, branched, nearly glabrous. Leaves sessile, lanceolate, acuminate, scabridly pubescent. Sheaths auricled. Spathes short-peduncled, broadly ovate-cordate. Petals white or blue. Seeds ellipsoid, straw coloured, puberulous. Racemes simple, 5-12-fid. Spathes longer than their peduncle, panicled or clustered.

Flowering: Rainy season

Distribution: Malay Islands, India and Nepal. Tropical India, from Nepal, Sikkim and Bengal in Central India, Madhya Pradesh and the Malay Peninsula.

Commelina paludosa Bl.

C. obliqua Buch-Ham. (non Vahl.)

C. obliqua Ham. (not of Vahl.)

Regional names: Kanjuna (Hindi), Kanjura (Hills-northern), Jatakanchura (Bengla)

Scandent or scrambling, perennial herbs. Stems branched from the base, decumbent or creeping and rooting below, suberect or ascending upwards, stout, subterete, glabrous. Leaves subsessile,lanceolate-oblong to oblong or elliptic-lanceolate, acuminate or acute, slightly oblique at base, scabrid 5-20 (-25) x 2-5 cm. Sheaths glabrous except a line of hairs, with an oblique ciliate mouth. Spathes subsessile or on 0.5-0.9 cm. long peduncles, 1-10 clustered at the ends of branches, funnel-shaped, with a cordate base, acuminate 1.5-2.3x2-3 cm. Cymes simple or branched once, on 1-1.5 cm. long peduncles. Pedicels 0.5-1.5 cm. long. Sepals unequal, dorsal one 0.3 cm. long; lateral ones 0.5 x 0.45-0.5 cm. Petals white, 0.6-0.7 cm. long. Staminodes 3, with 4-celled, stipitate anthers. Capsule 3-celled or rarely 2-celled, 3-seeded, 0.5 x 0.5 cm. Seeds ovoid-oblong, smooth, 0.4 x 0.25-0.3 cm.

Flowering: August-November

Distribution: Throughout India and in the hilly regions of Himalayas from the base or foot hills upto 6,000 ft. elevation regions.

Commelina undulata R.Br.

Family: Commelinaceae

C. kurzii Clarke

C. undulata R.Br. (excl. var. *setosa*) Rolla Rao

Perennial much branched, trailing, ascending or decumbent herb, with 30-70 cm. long, bracts, stems slender and thick, teret, glabrous. Leaves 4.7-12.5 x 1.6-5 cm., lanceolate, entire along margins, minutely hirsutulous and dark green above, glabrous and greyish green or somewhat stramceous below, acuminate at apex, rounded or suddenly contracted at base. Sheaths 1-2.5 cm. long, loose, striate, minutely hirtellus, ciliolate along margins at mouth. Spathes 2-5, terminal accompanied by 2-4 smaller leaves, each 1.7-2.5 cm. in diam., funnel-shaped, beaked on the anterior side peduncles 3-5 mm. long, covered by leaf-sheaths. Flowers in bifid cymes; inner clusters represented by stumps, outer 3-6 flowered. Sepals 3, membranous. Petals 3, violet or purplish violet, equal or subequal, clawed. Capsules 2-3 in. each spathe, each 5-6 cm. long oblong, 3-celled, 3-valved, each cell with free seed. Seeds about 5 mm. long, oval, greyish-black with a white membranous margin.

Flowering and fruiting: November-July

Plant occurring in the Upper Gangetic Plains, Siwaliks, U.P., Dehradun; Delhi and other several areas.

Commelina kurzii Cl.

A straggling or erect, tall herb, 60-90 cm. tall. Leaves 10-15x2-3 cm., variable, lanceolate, scabrous or villous; sheaths 2-5 cm. long, the mouth bearded. Spathes sessile, 2-2.5 x 1.5-2 cm., nearly as broad as long, crowded in terminal heads, scabrous. Flowers violet-blue. Capsules 3-celled; cells 1-seeded. Seeds smooth, lead-coloured.

Flowering and fruiting: August-October

Plant found in moist, shady places in gardens and lawns, also in plateaus, spreading upon rocked and growing in the cervices of stones; Delhi area and adjoining region.

Commelina ensifolia R.Br.

C. undulata var. *setosa* C.B. Clarke.

Family: Commelinaceae

Rhizomatous, diffuse, slender herbs. Leaves lanceolate, acute or acuminate, 7-9 x 0.5-1 cm. with sheath 2 cm. Flowers blue. Ovary 3-locular. Capsule 3-seeded.

Distribution: North Australia, Indis and Srilanka. Frequent in partial shade and in sandy terrain of plains, Karnataka; Tamilnadu, Deccan Peninsula, Southern India.

Commelina ensifolia Br. syn. *C. stricta* Wall (in part), *C. lunata* Heyne, *C. striataeaffinis* Edgw.

Stem 12-18 in., slender. Leaves 2-4 by 1/6-1/3 in., glabrous or with deciduous hairs, or villous. Spathes 1/2-2/3 in., glabrous or hairy, base truncate on one margin, hooked at the other raceme simple.

Deccan Peninsula, Southern India. Plant flowers in July to September.

Commelina paludosa Blume

C. obliqua Ham. ex D.Don.

C. polyspatha Wight.

Stout subscandent herbs upto 1 m. Leaves ovate to elliptic lanceolate, acuminate, often oblique at base, 10-16 x 4 cm. with rufous hairs at mouth and margin. Flowers blue. Ovary 3-locular. Seeds smooth, 1 per locule.

Indomalaysia. Occasional in shade of middle to upper Ghats and other places, Karnataka, Southern India. Plant flowers in August to December.

Commelina paludosa Blume.

Erect or ascending herbaceous plant, with broad lanceolate leaves with sheathing bases, and with flowers with 3 conspicuous pale blue to whitish petals, the flowers borne in the axils of obliquely funnel-shaped leafy bracts. Flowers

c. 8 mm. across; petals ovate, stalked; filaments of stamens hairless, bracts 2-3.5 cm. Leaves usually 5-10 cm., with basal sheaths fringed with hairs; stem sparsely branched 20-60 cm., rooting at the lower nodes.

Pakistan to South-West China, India, Burma, South-East Asia; Areas between 300 to 3500 m. elevation; Waste grounds, edges of cultivation, shrubberies. Plant flowers during the period form June to August.

Commelina kurzii Clarke

C. longifolia Thwaites (non Lamk.)

C. communis, C. striata Wall. (in part)

C. angustifolia Hassk.

Plant in Southern Deccan Peninsula, Malabar, and the Nilgiris Ceylon.

Commelina hasskarlii Clarke

C. salicifolia var. *brevifolia* Herb.

C. communis Wall. (in part)

Family: Commelinaceae

Decumbent-ascending, annual-perennial herbs. Stems branched from the base, creeping and rooting below, subterete, glabrous, upto 45-100 cm. high. Leaves subsessile, lanceolate oblong or elliptic-oblong, with a rounded base, subobtuse or subacute, scabrid on the margins, glabrous, up to 4-10x2-3 cm. Sheaths with an oblique mouth, ciliate, 1.5-2 cm. long. Spathes on 1.5-2 cm. long peduncles, ovate-lanceolate, acute, mucronate, glabrous, 3.5-4 x 1.5-2 cm. Cymes with lower 1-flowered branch and 2-flowered upper one, on 0.8-1 cm. long peduncles. Peduncles 0.2 cm. long. Outer tepals unequal, ovate, obtuse, 0.3 x 0.2-0.25 cm., inner ones blue. Capsule 5-celled, apiculate, glabrous, 0.8-1 x 0.4 cm. Seeds dark grey, smooth, 0.28-0.3 x 0.2 cm.

Flowering and fruiting: September-November

Distribution: Upper Gangetic Plains, Uttar Pradesh hills, and from Delhi eastward to Assam and Bengal, southward to the Deccan Peninsula. From Mt. Abu south to Konkan and Poona, Maharastra.

Commelina hasskarlii Cl.

A glabrous or pubescent, much-branched herb. Leaves narrowly lanceolate. Spathes-axillary, ovate-lanceolate, cordate, at the base. Flowers in pubescent, unequal cymes, the lower branch 1 to 2-flowered, upper 2 to 4-flowered. Capsules quadrate, apiculate. Seeds cylindric.

Plant occurring from Delhi to North Oudh, Siwaliks Upper Gangetic Plains, Siwaliks and foothills common in watersides and marshy, grassy localities.

Commelina forskalii Vahl.

C. falcata Hassk.

Family: Commelinaceae

Stem diffuse, rooting at the nodes. Leaves 1-2 by 1/4-1/2 in., narrowed at the base, margins often undulate. Spathes 1/2 in. broader than long, often hispid, base cuneate, or broadly truncate. Petals blue. Seeds lead-coloured, appendage O. Leafless suckers bear deformed capsules that ripen underground. Leaves glabrate, leaves sessile narrowly oblong, obtuse, spathes ovate or orbicular, shortly peduncled complicate or hooded acute, capsule with the lateral cells 0-1-seeded, dorsal striate, seeds subglobose smooth.

Flowering and fruiting: August-November

Distribution: Deccan Peninsula, Konkan.

Commelina forskalii Vahl. Regional names: Kankaua, Kana Diffuse, branched, creeping or straggling herb with serial chasmogamous and underground cleistogamous flowers, rooting at the nodes. Leaves linear or narrowly oblong, often undulate. Aerial spathes axillary, 3 to 5-flowered; flowers sky-blue. Capsule usually 3-seeded. Seeds smooth, subglobose. Cleistogamous flowers usually solitary in a spathe, bisexual, reduced. Capsules usually 1-seeded

Distribution: Deccan Peninsula, Konkan. Northern India plains; common on the ridges in sandy depressions, amonst stones, in the shades of shrubs; also found in fields, gardens and waste places; Delhi region, Haryana and adjacent zone, plant becoming abudant in patches in the provinces of northern parts.

Commelina subulata Roth.

C. *striata*

C.suburantiaca Hoechst.

Tradescantha triflora Heyne.

Family: Commelinaceae

Stem erect from a fibrous root, simple or branched. Leaves 1-3 by 1/10-1/4 in., acuminate, lips often hooked, usually glabrous or villously ciliate. Spathes 1/4 in long, scattered or clustered, acute, pubescent, base cordate. Flowers small, orange-purple or violet. Capsules 2 on each raceme, small, 3-5-seeded, dorsal valve at length 2-partite. Seeds puberulous, deeply transeveresly grooved.

Flowering and fruiting: August-October

Distribution: Deccan Peninsula

Commelina subulata Roth. Slender herbs, branching from base. Leaves linear-laneolate, acute, 10x0.5 cm. Spathes very small subsessile ovate-lanceolate falcate complicate. Flowers orange-coloured. Ovary 3-locular. Capsule 3-5-seeded.

Plant occurring in Southern India; Karnataka, common in open marshy soil of plains; Tamilnadu, Deccan Peninsula. Tropical Africa, India.

Genus *Commelina* Linnaeus in the family Commelinaceae (about 230 tropical and subtropical species; genera 25 with species nearly 300; tropical and subtropical) with salient features.

Herbs usually slender or creeping below. Leaves ovate-lanceolate or linear with lax sheaths, petioled or not. Flowers in usually 2-fid, cymes emerging one at a time from a terminal complicate or funnel-shaped or hooded spathe; flowers of the upper cyme-branch small, deciduous, of the lower fertile; fruiting pedicel and capsule retrated within the spathe. Sepals 3, membranous, the 2 inner often connate at the base. Petals 3, longer than the sepals, one larger than the others and often clawed. Stamens 3, perfect, with 2-3 imperfect; anthers oblong, one usually longer than the others. Ovary 3-rarely 2-celled, two of the cells 1 or 2-ovuled, thrid cells, if present, 1-ovuled or empty. Fruit a loculicidal capsule hidden in the spathe by the decurving of the pedicel after flowering, the posticuous cell indehiscent and connate as a ligulate body, from which the posterior cell fall away. Seeds ellipsoid or angled; testa reticulate pitted or rugose.

Genus *Commelina* Linn. with about 230 species in tropical and subtropical regions, and 23 species in India; chiefly in Southern and Western India and a few occur throughout India (family Commelinaceae with about 38 genera and 500 species and 10 genera and 76 species in India, chiefly in Southern and Western India and tropical Eastern Himalaya).

Genus *Commelina* in tries II Commelineace (in family Commelinaceae) having capsule loculicidal and 2 perfect stamens with 1-3 staminodes, has specifically cymes solitary included in a spathe and ovary 3-celled with 1-2-ovuled cells in *Commelina*, and separates from genus *Aneilema* R.Br. Other genera of Commelinaceae particularly *Cynotis* Don. and *Floscopa* Lour. have 6 perfect or fertile stamens, and capsule loculicidal (in tribe III with other genera also). *Commelina* genus is with 4-6 stamens, with 3 fertile ones and 1-3 staminodes; and further *Commelina* with inflorescence not paniculate and bracts spathaceous differs from *Murdannina* Royle having inflorescence a cymose panicle and bracts not spatahecous. Broadly the family Commelinaceae comprises epiphytic as well as terrestrial plants, and the genus *Commelina* belongs to later habitat and leaf sheaths not inflated. Two genera *Commelina* and *Cynotis* have a cyme inflorescence but *Commelina* is distinguished of floral bracts inconspicous and presence of staminodes. Various species of *Commelina* Linn. are distinguishable by their specific characterstics of different parts of these plants. *Commelina benghalensis* Linn. has ovate leaves with obtuse or rounded tips and 5-seeded capsule; whereas other *Commelina paludosa* Blume. has lanceolate leaves with acute tip and 3-seeded capsule.

The characters of spathe separate *Commelina diffusa* N. Burm. from other species. Peduncle of spathe long about 2-3 cm. and spathe folded in middle in *Commelina diffusa;* whereas some other species of *Commelina* are with peduncle of spathe hardly 1 cm. or none and funnel-shaped spathe.

The under ground stems and ovary differ in two species. *Commelina benghalensis* has underground stem with bulb-like cleistogamous flowers and 2-locular ovary; whereas the underground stem without cleistogamous flowers and 3-locular ovary are in *Commelina paludosa.* This species is further distinguished for robust plant, with leaves up to 10x5 cm. from another species *Commelina subulata* Roth of slender plants. with leaves up to 10x1.5 cm. *Commelina subulata* Roth. has spathe recurved in perennial plants in dry compacted soil; whereas spathe is erect in the annual plants of *Commelina ensifolia* R.Br. in wet sandy soils.

On the basis of organs and other characters of ovary mainly the species are separated. All the cells of ovary 1-ovuled and smooth seeds are in *Commelina kurzii* Cl.; and in some others species, the two anticous cells of ovary 2-ovuled and the posticous 1-ovuled. Structure of leaves and characters of seeds differ in these species. Leaves usually ovate, broader and seeds rugose in *Commelina benghalensis* L.; whereas lanceolate and narrower leaves and smooth, truncate at one end seeds are in two species of *Commelina* but they differ for spathe, ovary and capsule characters. *Commelina forskalii* Vahl. has ovate and broad spathe, 5-ovuled ovary but usually 3-seeded capsules and posticous cells not keeled; whereas spathe ovate-lanceolate, capsules usually 5-seeded and posticous cells keeled in *Commelina hasskarlii* Cl.

In general the plant *Commelina benghalensis* Linn. is very variable in habit, hairiness, size and shape of leaves. The flowers colour sometimes in *Commelina paludosa* Bl. is blue, but they are white, petals pale blue, one or them nearly white or sky blue in other plants of different areas; and the flowers in this species are with 3 conspicous pale blue to whitish petals in variations practically.

Commelina tuberosa Linn. syn. *Commelina coelestis* Willd. Erect herb, 25-46 cm. high, roots more orless tuberous, branches with clasping, long broad-lanceolate, pointed leaves 7.5 x 15 cm. long, minutely scabrous or glabrous. Spathes pubescent, rounded or cordate at base, with wavy margins, spathe leaves, ovate, folded, sheaths ciliate, upper racemes 4-10 flowered, lower 1-2 flowered, hairy, two minor sepals slightly connate; petals deep blue, about 1.5 cm. long.

Plant native of Mexico and running wild. Siwaliks, Dehradun (Mussorie) and other areas.; descending upto 800 m. alt. localities. Plant flowers and fruits during the rainy seasons.

Two species *Commelina tuberosa* Linn. and *Commelina coelestis* Willd. are considered hardly distinct and become synonymous. Another species *Commelina forskalaei* Vahl. is apparently distinguished from *Commelina benghalensis* Linn. by its linear leaves and smooth seeds. In case of *Commelina paludosa* Bl., besides the flowers colour blue or white, the plant has short-peduncled spathes add in the occasional presence of 2-celled capsules.

The leaves, roots and whole plant of *Commelina benghalensis* Linn. are medicinally useful.

Plant is bitter, emollient, demulcent, refrigerant, laxative, and benefecial in leprosy.

Leaves are useful in fever, scorpion sting, wounds, and other ailments. Whole plant is useful as laxative, and refrigerant. Roots are useful in liver complaints. Roots are used in fever. Whole plant is considered useful in snake bite and sores. Leaves are used as vegetable and preparing 'Pakorhas' (dish prepared with gram flour or Besan and fried in cooking oil media usually) which are relished.

Leaves are eaten by poor people as a pot-herb, especially in times of scarcity. Fleshy rhizomes of some of the species of genus contain much starch mixed with mucilage, and they are whole some food when cooked.

The juice of flowers was used as a bluish pigment in painting upon transparencies.

The leaves, roots and whole plant of *Commelina diffusa* Burm. f. syn. *Commelina nudiflora* Linn. are medicinally useful.

Bruised herb is applied to burns, itches and boils. Leaves are used for applying poultice over sores.

Roots are useful in fever, biliousness and as an antidote to snake bite.

The roots, leaves and whole plant of *Commelina paludosa* Bl. syn. *Commelina obliqua* Buch.-Ham. are medicinally useful.

Roots are considered an antidote to snake poison, and useful in vertigo, fever and bilious affections. Roots are laxative and refrigerant.

Whole plant of *Commelina paludosa* Bl. are useful in insects sting, and some other ailments.

The plant *Commelina suffruticosa* Bl. is medicinally useful. It is considered useful in menorrhagia. Roots are applied to sores.

Whole plant of *Commelina salicifolia* Roxb. is useful in dysentery and insanity.

Medicinal properties and actions of the plant drug-Rasa Tikta-kaṣāya-madhura, Vīrya sīta, Vipāka kaṭu, Pitta hara, Guṇa rūkṣa-lalghu, sita; Karma Grāhi, Stambhana, Rucya, Sāraka, Kaṇḍūghna, Viṣabhna, Dāhaprasamana, Jvaraghna, Vraṇa-ropaṇa, Vimlāpana, Pittasaṁsamana, and Snehana; and therapeutic indications of internal and external uses in Jvara, Kaṇḍu, Visphoṭa, Vraṇa, Sotha, Viṣa, Sarpadaṁsa, Vṛscikadamsa, Yakrdvikāra, Pittavikāra, Agnidagdh, Dāha, Koṣṭha-baddhatā and other diseases.

Kaṅcaṭa, Karṇapatra, the Sanskrit names for plant drug.

Kaṅcaṭa: Kaiyadeva Nighaṇṭu, Auṣadhi varga, 731

8

Costus speciosus (Koenig.) Sm.

Costus speciosus var. *nepalensis* (Rosc.) Baker.

Banksia speciosa Keenig.

Family: Costaceae (Scitaminaceae/Zingiberaceae)

Regional names: Keu (Hindi), Chunnak-koova (Malayalam), Keu (Bengla); Penva (Marathi), Kemuka (Bombay) Kuravam (Tamil), Chengalva-koshtu (Telgu & Kannarease); Kust, Besemaṭi, Keukanda, Chana, Keokanda; Kottam; Kostam (Tamil), Kashmeeramu (Telgu).

Erect herbaceous plant, 4-6 ft. high, Stem somewhat wooly at the base. Leaves subsessile, arranged spirally, 8-12 in. long, oblong or oblanceolate, acute or acuminate, often cuspidate, glabrous above, silky pubescent beneath, base rounded, sheaths coriaceous; ligule none. Flowers many, in dense terminal spikes 2-5 in. long; bracts bright red, ovate, acuminate or pungently mucronate, bracteoles solitary calyx deltoid-ovate, cuspidate; corolla-tube as long as the calyx, lobes ovate-oblong, apiculate, lateral lobes longer and dorsal one rather shorter; lip suborbicular, white with a yellow centre, 2 in. or more in diam, concave, plicate, crisped, disk pubescent with a tuft of hairs at the base; stamens with a tuft of hairs of the base of the filament, connective petaloid, about 1/2 in. broad, pubescent, produced into two glabrous appendages about as long as the linear anther-cells; style slender, about 1.5 in. long; stigma with a semilinear ciliate mouth. Capsule small, globosely trigonous, red. Seeds black, with a white aril.

Flowering and fruiting:	Flowers during the rainy season. August-September, October-November
Distribution:	Outer ranges of Himalaya upto 4,500 ft. alt., more or less throughout India; Bengal, Kashmir and Uttar Pradesh. Often cultivated as an ornamental plant. Ceylon, Malaya Peninsula and Islands, and also in China.

Plant occurring wild particularly in Bengal, Kashmir and also in Uttar Pradesh; Siwalik ranges, common in Sal forests and southwards along the Sub-Himalayan tracts of Bundelkhand and north Oudh, usually in moist shady places and also other localities; and abundantly in areas as Bengal and Kashmir, and other provinces in country.

Costus speciosus (Koenig ex Retz.) E. Smith. syn. *Banksia speciosa* Koenig. ex Retz.

Erect, perennial herbs, with a tuberous, horizontal, rhizomatous rootstock. Stems up to 3 cm. tall, clothed with sheaths in the lower part, leafy upwards. Leaves subsessile oron 0.3-0.7 cm. long petioles, obovate-oblanceolate to oblong, acuminate-caudate, glabrous and dark green above, appressed-pubescent on the lower surface, white margined, ciliate 15-35 X 6-10 cm. sheaths upto 4 cm. long, with an obliquely truncate hairy mouth, ciliate. Inflorescence an ovoid-oblong, 3-10 cm. long, slightly curved spike. Bracts, lanceolate-oblong, cuspidate, ciliate, glabrate, 2.5-4 x 1-1.5 cm. Bracteoles red, lanceolate, keeled, 1-2 cm. long. Calyx 2-2.5 cm. long, glabrous, sub 2-lipped; 2 posterior lobes ovate-triangular, 0.5-0.7 cm. long, anterior one lanceolate, apiculate, 1 cm. long. Corolla-tube 0.5-0.7 cm. long, lobes obovate-oblanceolate, apiculate, 4.5-5 x 1.5-2 cm. Lip trumpet-shaped, white, crispy-serrate, with a yellowish, hairy throat, hairy along the median creamy band, 5-6 cm. across.

Staminodes O; filament hairy on the back, 3-4 cm. long. Style 4-5 cm. long; stigma with a semi-lunar, ciliate mouth. Capsule 3-gonous, bright red.

Plant commonly occurring in forest edges, forest clearings, sal forests and ravine slopes in Siwaliks, Dehradun, U.P.

Costus speciosus (Koenig.) Smith. Flowers white, funnel-shaped with contrasting large bright red bracts, numerous in a very dense cylindrical spike 5-10 cm. long, borne on a stout red leafy stem 1-2 m. Flowers c. 4 cm.; bracts ovate, 1.5-4 cm. long. Calyx with 3 oval lobes; corolla-tube shorter than calyx, with un equal petals 2.5-4 cm., lip white with an orange red centre, rounded, 5-8 cm., forming a funnel with margins incurved and meeting. Leaves oblong acute, sheathing at base, 15-30 cm. Capsule red, crowned with persistent calyx.

Uttar Pradesh to Sikkim, India. Burma; upto 1500 m. alt. in Himalayan ranges, forests, shrubberies. Plant in Flowering stage during the period June to August.

Costus speciosus is a perennial herb surviving through the branched rhizomes. Its aerial stem, usually straight and unbranched, perishes in autumn and fresh sprouts reappear in the following spring.

The cultivation of the plant *Costus speciosus* (Koem.) Sm. for procurement of rhizome is taken up which is the commercially important part of plant which has certain nut ritional requirement as fertiliser amendments with essential nutrients for its systematic and productive yield in farming on large scale and also experimental purpose. The active constituents of the plant is diosgenin which is an important raw material for synthesis of various steroidal drugs as well as medicinal utility as raw drug.

Distribution: Java, Malacca

Costus kingii Baker. Leaves pubescent, beneath, peduncle longer produced direct from the rootstock, bracts-leaves larger oblong, corolla villous.

Leaves 6-8 by 3-3.5 in., oblanceolate-oblong, subcoriaceous branched above the middle, narrowed gradually to the base. Peduncle 4-5 in., stout; bracts 2 in., densely imbricate, oblong, scariose. Spike 2.5-3 in., very dense, globose; outer bracts above, in., ovate; linear lanceolate. Calyx tube 1 in., villous, segments ovate, sharply cuspidate. Corolla-segments 1 in., hairy. Lip suborbicular 2 in long and broad.

Distribution: Perak, Larut

Costus speciosus (Koenig.) Smith

Costus speciosus Sm.

Costus arabicus Jacq.

Costus speciosus var. *nipalensis* Rosc.

Hellenia grandiflora Retz.

Costus speciosa var. *argyrophyllus* Wall.

Banksia speciosa Koenig.

Tall, rarely branching herbs, with creeping tuberous rootstock and twisting stem with spiralling foliage cm. Roots stocks tuberous, horizontal. Leafy stem long. Leaves elliptic obovate, white-pubescent beneath. Bracts of inflorescence bright-red; calyx red, lobes ending in a hardened prickle; at centre. Seeds globose in capsule 1 in, globose, red.

Indomalaysia; fairly common across Ghats, Karnataka. Throughout India from Central and Eastern Himalayas (ascending to 4,000 ft. alt.) to Ceylon and Malacca; Malay Islands; Burma, Pegu and Penang.

The procurement plant *Costus speciosus* (Koen.) Sm. for the rhizone may be made from commercially important part of plant through cultivation for various requirements.

The fertiliser supplements with essential nutrients for its systematic and productive yield in farming on large scale and also experimental purpose. The active constituents of the plant is diosgenin which is an important raw material for synthesis of various steroidal drugs as well as medicinal utility as raw drug.

It is estimated (CROMAP, 14-2, 123, 1992) that maximum rhizome yield of 34.52 tons/hac and maximum crude diosgenin 47/61 kgs/has is obtained under the combination treatment of N 150 kgs/has, $P_2 O_2$ 100 kgs/has and K_3 O 100 kgs/hac. The crude diosgenin yield varies from 0.63 to 0.74% in solution culture by 16 meq. of P and 4 meq of K. The maximum yield is obtained by 80 kg N/hac with 30X60 cm spacing. The proportion for mixing these fertilisers in ratio 40:40:40 NPK kgs/hac is considered best for good yield of *Costus* rhizomes through higher productivity.

The roots are important part of the plant. Rhizomes or tubers are medicinally useful. Roots are bitter, astringent, stimulant, digestive, anthelmintic, depurative and aphrodisiac. These are useful in catarrhal fevers, cough, dyspepsia, worms, skin diaseases and snake-bite. Tubers are cooked and made into a syrup or preserve which is considered very wholesome.

Medicinal properties and actions of the drug-Rasa tikta, madhura kaṭu, Vīrya Uṣṇa, Vipāka kaṭu, Guṇa, laghu; and kāntiprada, sukrala, kaṇḍūghna, kuṣṭhaghna, jvraghna, viṣaghna, meghana kāsaghna, svāsāghna, kaṇṭhya, viṣarpahara, vātaraktahara, dīpana, rocana, hṛdya, grāhī, raktavikārahara; Kaphapittahara and vātavardhaka. Its potent medicinal properties and action mainly include its Garbhāsaya saṅkocaka karma.

Therapeutic indications and uses in cardiac diaorders, urinary anomalies, lepratic diseases, fever, cough, asthma, seminal complaints, blood impurities and complaints, vertigo, Agnimāndya or gastric troubles and other complaints.

The rhizome and other parts such as stems, leaves and whole plant are used in medicinal and allied purposes. Various applications of this plant drug made in different kinds of ailments carry internal and external modes of administration in several recipes.

Roots or rhizomes are used in anasarca, bodyache, cough, asthma, bronchitis, cold, cholera, constipation, dropsy, dysentery, giddiness, jaundice, leprosy, pthisis, stomach troubles, general debility, overthirst, heat sensation, indigestion, worms, stomach troubles and diarrhoea. Plant considered useful in dog bite or rabid. Stems is useful for burn cases as external application, and also used as maggotcidal plant. Leaves are applied in scabies and other similar skin affections. Roots are considered useful in postnatal care. Leaves are topically applied to wounds and ulcers. Rhizome is useful as galactogogue medicine and bilary troubles and as cooling medicine. Rhizomes are considered useful in eye and ear complaints. Roots are anthelmintic and used in worms troubles. Rhizomes are useful as stimulant medicine.

Rhizomes of the plant are also edible and employed or consumed in different forms like pickles, vegetable, drinks and other similar articles. It has aromatic value for its use as perfumery plant substance.

The pharmacological activity of the plant shows that the saponins in drug plant have significant anti-inflammatory and anti-arthritic activities against acute pedal inflammation induced by carrageenin (1 per cent) and formalin (1 percent) in albino rats. It also significantly suppresses the inflammatory exudate formation in croton oil granuloma pouch and granulation tissue formation by cotton pellet implantation in albino rars. The results compared with betamethazone are qualitatively similar though less effective but with the advantage of not producing gastric lesions common with corticosteroids.

The total saponins mixture show significant anti-inflammatory activity; and the results compared quantitatively with those obtained with betamethazone. The saponins increase significantly weight of uterus in sprayed albino rats, and the results being comparable to those produced by stilboesterol. The saponins produce proliferative changes in the uterus and vagina which is similar to those produced by stilboesterol.

The plant is pharmacologically quite active as potential drug in uterine activity. The comparative study of the uterine activity of *Costus speciosus* and *Gloriosa superba* finds that the fresh juice of both the plants has a stimulant action on isolated preparation of guinepigs, rabbit and dog's uterus in situ. The plant *Costus* has a stimulant action on isolated rat uterus, whereas *Gloriosa* has a papaverine-like action. Thus the plant *Costus speciosa* is found to be 2-3 times more potent than *Gloriosa superba* as an ecoblic phytoagent. The ecbolic activity of *Costus speciosus)* is found in chloroform extract (containing saponins as a most potent ecbolic agent exerting its action directly on the uterine muscle on the basis of effect found on isolated estrinized rat's uterine.

The effect of plant on uterus and other reproductive organs has been studied biologically through animal and human experimentations. The crops of five saponins of the chloroform extract have been studied individually on estrinzized rat uterus. The mother residue, and crop B seems to be inert, crop A very mild relaxant, crop C very mild stimulant and crop D, E and F strong agents. Detailed studies of crop D in rat, guineapig, rabbit and dog and also human uterus, in different hormonal conditions viz. diestrus, melestrus and estrus phases, oestrogen and progester one treated uterus and puerperal stage, as well as different stages of pregrancy and also in situ preparations reveal about its strong direct stimulation or stimulant action on the uterus. The relaxant effect is observed on the human fallopian tube, isolated human uterus, pregnant uteri and uteri in situ of guineapig, rabbit and dog seemed to be highly sensitive to its stimulant action specially on the uterus as phyto stimulant and ecbolic agent.

The observations of studies on ovariectomised albino rates by injecting plant extract on consecutive five days and compared with those receiving only oestrogen for five days and another group receving oestrogen for five day followed by the plant extract for another five days. The extract-treated rats show marked proliferation and cornification of vaginal epithelium comparable with that found in the estrous phase in ovariectomised rats. The third group receiving both oestrogen and the plant extract, certification of vaginal epithelium shows the absence and with little proliferation. It is hormonal effect and plant extract activity particularly their mutual observation on uterus and allied organs.

The alkaloids isolated from the plant possess anti-cholinesterase activity both in vitro and in vivo confirming the earlier observations of potentiation of acetycholine responses on frog rectus muscle and dog blood pressure. The alkaloids like physostigmine almost equally effective against true and pseudo-cholinesterase, but prove much weaker than physostigmine. In addition the use of the plant in eye diseases and as a depurative might be due to its anticholinesterase activity found in the alkaloidal contents of drug.

In general the pharmacology of plant covers various active principles or compounds and alkaloids present in the plant i.e. rhizome, and the pharmacological activities are due to different chemical contents isolated from the plant drug. For the instance, the saponins are responsible for pasmolytic, cardiovascular, haemolytic, anti-inflammatory and anti-arthritic activity of drug. Diosgenin have estrogenic effect. Rhizomes have action on uterine muscles resulting into ecbolic activity, anticholinesterase, anti-inflammatory and effect on vagina of ovarietcomised rats.

Pharmacognostically the rhizomes of *Costus speciosus* (Koen.) Sm. are found adulterated with rhizomes of different plant *Gloriosa superba* Linn. (Liliaecae) in various parts of the northern India. The salient features of roots and rhizomes of these two plant differ on the basis of macro and microscopic characterstics. Mainly the rhizomes *Costus* are cylindrical or slightly flattened with bitter taste, and fibres remain absent, whereas the rhizomes of *Gloriosa* are tuberous and inspid, with fibres. Vascular bundles in *Costus* are collateral with slight extensions of phloem on both sides of xylem, when the vascular bundles in *Gloriosa* are almost surrounded by xylem or amphicrebal. In the rhizomes of *Costus* the starch grains show concentrace striations, and these do not show striations and shorter in measurement in the rhizomes of *Gloriosa* comparatively.

The roots of these two plants also carry difference in the salient characterstics. Chiefly the cork cambium arises in the first layes of cortex and forms three parts of or layers cork cells in *Costus,* whereas the cork cambium in *Gloriosa* arises in the third layer of cortex, by forming 3 to 5 layers of cork cells. The central portion of the wood in *Costus* after lignffication becomes delignified to a large extent, the roots of *Gloriosa* show only small delignification. In the roots of *Costus* the cortical aprenchyma gets disintegrated forming air-spaces, but no such disintegration occurs in the roots of *Gloriosa* plant.

The rhizomes of *Gloriosa superba* are adulterants of *Costus speciosus* carrying pharmacognostic and pharmacologicol resemblance distinctions and comparative features. The chemical screening finds that tigogenin and diosgenin in the free state are isolated from the petroleum ether extract of dried rhizomes of *Costus speciosus.* The chloroform extract of the deflated rhizomes yields a mixture of five saponins as revealed by TLC as only one saponin, glucoside of B-sitosterol and other compound, could be isolated in pure crystalline form. The saponin mixture on acid hydrolysis exhibited the presence of four sapogenins in different proportions by TLC and only B-sitosterol and diosgenin could isolated from plant, another sapogenins present in traces remained inseparable. The alocoholic extract of the dried rhizomes on acid hydrolysis yielded 3.86 per cent total sapogenin yielded about 2.12 per cent pure diosgenin on further crystallisation and chromatography. The diosgenin content is compared favourably with that of *Dioscorea prazeri*.

In the chloroform extract of the dried powdered rhizomes of *Costus speciosus*, the two saponias are isolated. Saponin A is isolated as granules with m.p. 289-290°, on acid hydrolysis gave glucose and B-sitosterol and saponin B also as granules having m.p. 305-307°, on acid hydrolysis yielded diosgenin, glucose and rhamose. The saponins A, B and C, differed from each other in the relative proportions of glucose and rhamonose revealed by chromotographic observations. Glucose dominated over harmones in three saponins.

The chemical profile of rhizome of the plant has occurrence of important contents of diosgenin (during 1970s). Its use as a raw material for the steroidal industry has been later emphasized, and a wide clonal variations in its crude diosgenin content ranging between 0.5% to 4.0%, and pure diosgenin; diosgenin upto 2.0% on dry weight basis. The rhizomes possess 15-20% dry matter and 80-85% moisture.

Chemically speaking this plant has come into prominence after the isolation of diosgenin from its rhizome in a yield of 2.12% as dry weight basis. The presence of free diosgenin and tigogenin in the rhizomes. Two saponins, dioscin and gracillin have been isolated from the rhizome. Diosgenin content and the presence of fatty acids in the seeds have also been further studied add observed that seeds 2 kgs. yielded 9.5 g. of sapoinin in the alcoholic extract and 1.3 g. diosgenin as genin. Seeds oil contain its major constituents such as oleic, palmitic, linoleic and stearic acids. Seeds are also found as an additional storage or source of diosgenin.

Two new compounds have been isolated from the roots of plant namely 24-hydroxy hentriacontan-27-one and hydrixytria contan-26-one by spectral data and chemical analysis. Some other compounds methylriacontaoate diosgenin and B-sitosterol from the roots of plant. A novel type of sterol possessing particular bond is also isolated 5a-stigmast.

The seeds of the plant are found to contain more saponins, as eight saponins isolated named constucoside A to H (with specific structures). Two more furostannol saponins named costucoside I and J. Further two new alphatic compounds are isolated and characterized from the roots as B-hydroxy-tricontan-25-one and MC-triacontanoate-25-32. Some new compounds B-sitosterol B-D-glucoside, prosapogenin B of dioscin, Prosapogenin A of dioscin and gracillin have been later isolated. Four compounds detected in the hexane extract of the roots which include two compounds identified as methyl hexadecanoate, and methyl octadecanoate. Another compounds isolated have been characterised as tetracosanyl octadecanoate.

Further five new compounds have been isolated which are identified as 13-methylpentadecanoate, tetradecyl 11-methyl-tridecanaote 14-exotricosanotic acid, 14-oxoheptacosanoic acid, and 14-oxoctacosaonic acid by spectral and chemical screening.

Other compounds Triacontanol 5a-stigmast-9, triacontanoic acid, sitosterol and diosgenin have also been isolated. Four triterpenes, 31-corcycloartanone, cyclooartenyl acetate and cyclonaudenyl acetate have been further identified.

As regards the biosythesis and translocation of diosgenin in the plant, radioactively labelled free and conjugated diosgenin has been isolated from different parts of plant such as stem, leaves, seeds, flowers and rhizomes. Percent distribution of radioactivity in various parts of *Costus speciosus* is suggested (i) diosgenin biosgenin is biosynthesized in leaves and then translocated to all the parts of plant, (ii) glycosidation of diosgenin taking place in all the parts of plant and disogenin glycosides stored in rhizomes, seeds and flowers, and (iv) deglycosidation of saponin observe only in the rhizome responsible for hydrolysis.

There is variability in diosgenin contents. Optimum conditions for harvesting and producing better yield of diosgenin have also the rhizomes has been for their different characters and diosgenin content for two successive generations. The diosgenin accumulates in seeds and rhizomes, whereas other parts of the plant act for translocation of diosgenin.

Diosgenin has been isolated from rhizomes, stems and flowers of other species of *Costus* such as *Costus arabicus, C. spiralis C. villarisimus, C. quanoiensis,* by capillary and preperative chromatography, NMR, IR and mass spectroscopy. Lanosterol, tigogenin, diosgenin, stigmasterol, B-sitosterol and costugenin have been isolated from *Costus afar.* Diosgenin is isolated in *Costus malorticanus* on dry weight basis in rhizomes, roots, stems and leaves, and this plant has become a new source for disogenin. The rhizomes of *Costus spiralis* contained 4 furastanol glycosides, which after hydrolysis yielded diosgenin, glucose and rhamnose.

Genetic studies on ploidy status, diosgenin contents, genotype and environment are made on *Costus speciosus.* Physiological observations are on effect of growth and respiratory regulators on diosgenin synthesis, split application of potassium on rhizome yield and diosgenin by *Costus speciosus*. Other relevant informations indicate about enzymatic transformation of glycosides, induced sprouting, post-harvest induced changes of diosgenin content, effect of rhizome diameter on sapogenin content, and effect of endogenous enzymes on disogenin content and allied data.

As regard the instrumental analysis, an HPLC method is followed for the determination of diosgenin content. Diosgenin is detected in the eluate by differential refractometry. Carbon 13-NMR spectral analysis of spirostanol and furostanol glycosides of *Costus speciosus* has been detected. A GLC method has been adopted for the estimation of diosgenin in the plant. Further capillary gas-liquid chromatographic determination method for estimation of diosgenin in the plant *Costus speciosus* has also been followed.

For the tissue culture of *Costus speciosus*, the unorganised culture of the plant, when fed with different concenrations of cholesteral showed a significant increase in diosgenin content. Disogenin content found low in differentiated cells; 0.15-0.48%). Two steroidal sapogenins are isolated from the rhizome and stem callyus of the plant *Costus speciosus* by thin-layer chromatography and identified as disogenin and tigogenin. Both sapogenins found present in all tissue samples analysed, except two week old stem Callus, in which trigogenin found absent. Physical and IR spectral data are observed. Diosgenin, trigogenin, lanosterol and stigmasterol are determined in callus cultures of *Costus speciosus* at different periods (weeks) of culturing the tissue samples of plant.

Maximum contents of diosgenin (0.71%), tigogenin (0.37%), and lanosterol (0.78%) found after 2 weeks. Callus of plant contained 1.08% sapogenin. Suspension cultures of *Costus* and some other plants i.e. certain species of *Solanam* and Dioscorea, after monitoring (with due transfer at room temperature liquid medium) for diosgenin formation showed increasement in all cultures fed with kinetin and sugar cane juice as compared with controls. The rhizomes and leaves of field grown plants contained 2.0 and 0.40% diosgenin respectively.

The chemical profile and its review (CROMAP, 10.4, 168-183, 1988) of the plant *Costus speciosus* covers about 30 compounds isolated from the rhizomes and other parts of plant i.e. roots and seeds mainly. These chemical constituents may broadly be put into following groups:

1. Sapogenin
2. Saponins
3. Sterols/Triterpene
4. Aliphatic compounds-Easters, Oxe acids and Branched

   Fatty Acid Easters, Fatty acids
5. Hydroxy Ketones
6. Benzoquinones
7. Tocopherol

Further, the studies on genetics and plant breeding specially on the mechanism of 2n pollen formation in diloids of *Costus speciosus* (Koenig) J.E. Smith and importance of sexual ply-ploidization in the origin of interspecific chromosomal races showed that the absence of cytokinesis detected in some of the dyads at the close of second meiotic division as the mechanism producing 2n pollen in both the diloids. Distinct variation in n and 2n pollen size indicated the possibility of its use forestimating the frequency of 2n pollen in large populations. The sexual polyploidization involving the function of 2n gammetes has important role in the origin of naturally occurring interspecific chromosomal races of the plant.

In addition, the methylester of para-coumaric acid has been identified as the antifungal principles of the rhizomes of *Costus speciosus* (Koen.) Sm.

Genus *Costus* in the family Zingiberaceae or popularly known as Ginger family (46 genera and 850 species in tropics, abundant in Indo-Malesia) has about 150 tropical species and one species occurs throughout India, ascending upto 1,320 m. in the Himalayas; some times considered as the type of a distinct family Costaceae.

Genus *Costus* Linnaeus (in the family Scitamiaceae-Zingiberaceae—Costaceae) with salient features-Perennial. tall, rarely branching herbs, with creeping tuberous root-stock and twisting stem to leaves appear spiralled. Leaves alternate, shortly petioled, simple; sheath tubular, closed, ligulate; venation striate. Inflorescence a dense terminal cone-like spike, with spirally arranged bracts. Flowers irregular, bisexual. Calyx tubular, 3-toothed. Corolla 3-lobed, flat forming one of the petioled structure. Stamens 1, the filament, together with the connective, forming an oblong petaloid process with contiguous, 2-celled, linear anther at its middle. Two staminodes combined in large, petaloid, suborbicular or obovate, marginally cuspid lip (labellum); other resembles minute or O. Ovary inferior, 2-tubular; ovules many, axile, style filiform, erect; stigma with a crescent-shaped depression, hairy at sides. Fruit a globose, irregularly dehiscing capsule, with many, shortly arillate seeds.

Salient characters of the genus *Costus* with leaves spirally arranged, with tubular sheaths; stamens with a broad, petaloid filaments which curves forwards with an upturned tip, whereas various other genera like *Catimbium* Juss., *Curcuma* Linn., *Globra* Linn., *Hedychium* Koenig ex Retz. and *Zingiber* Boehm. have generally leaves distichous, with sheaths open on the side opposite to the lamina; and other specific characters of flowers and their organs in different genera distinctively.

In view of the Himalayan genera, the genus *Costus* Linn. has leaves spirally arranged and the leaf-sheaths tubular, closed; whereas other genera such as *Curcuma, Roscoea, Cautleya* and *Hedychium* are with leaves in 2 ranks and the leaf-sheath open one side in general, and further differing for various floral characterstics.

Genus *Costus* Linn. in family Costaceae comprisning *Costus speciosus* specifically with leaves elliptic-obovate, upto 30x8 cm., glabrous above, white-pubescent beneath are distinguishing.

The plant is useful in perfumery. It appears to be scarcely as odorous as Orris roots. The tincture has an aggreable smell, and would be useful, but no quantity might has as yet been seen in the market. An unlimited quantity might easily enough be compared from Bengal were some effort made to bring this root before the perfumers of Europe. The rhizomes of Costus are also reported to be substitute or aduletarant of roots of *Saussurea lappa* C.B. Clarke. (Asteraceae) which is botanical source of a major drug Kuṣṭha.

The root stock was said to be used as a substituted for the ginger. The rhizomes of *Costus* resembles the great Galangal in growth and structure, but has no aromatic properties, the taste being mucilaginous and feebly astringent, it could only be used as substitute for ginger by being preserved with a quantity of that root was eaten by tribals, and root sufficient to flavour it.

The *Costus* or kust root was given as a depurative and aphrodisiac. There seems no doubt for earlier using or considering it as *Saussurea* or Kuth, but that a certain amount of the tubers of *Costus speciosus* are regularly used by the natives of India as food and medicine.

Simhaless natives were using this drug as a medicine in rhizome form. In north-western provinces, a strengtheing tonic was prepared from the roots which was also used as anthelmintic. Some tribals or rural native were prescribing the rhizomes of this plant for alleviating the pain in marrow. The admission that it was used medicinally in the Concan confirms the general line adopted; the kust of the drug shops was often most probable not *Costus* but *Saussurea,* but for some unexplainable reason the roots of these plants had been confused, and in literature on the subject, there was no resemblance to each other, perhaps for the past 200 years, but at the same time there was a view about certain amount of *Costus specious* root deliberately used and not from any idea of adulteration with the supposed *Costus* of the ancients.

Kemuka: Kaiyadeva Nighaṇṭu, Oṣadhi Nighaṇṭu, 1607-1609; Synonymy for Kemuka or Sanskrit terms: Kemuka, Pelu, Pecula, Peluni and Dalasālinī; op. cit., 1607

9

Leonotis nepetifolia (L.) R.Br.

Leonotis nepetaefolia Br.

Phlomis nepetaefolia Linn.

Leonurus globosus Moench.

Family: Lamiaceae (Labiatae)

Regional names: Hejurchet (Bengla), Matijer (Bombay), Ranabheri (Telgu), Janvan dhompa (Santals), Ranabheri, beri, mulu gonamidu hau umatabira (Telgu), Mahayagmar, assa (Singa.), Dipamal (Marathi), Hejurchei (Hindi), Matijer, matisul (Gujarati), Dare dhompo, Janam dhompo (Santal); Barchibuti, Dhompo, Gogadkusir, Mota-shool Bara-guma

Erect, annual herbs. Stems obtusely 4-angular, deeply grooved, puberulous. Leaves ovate, acute, create-serrate with a cuneate base. Verticillasters in dense spikes. Bracts spine-tipped. Calyx prominently ribbed, hairy, tube incurved, with an oblique mouth, teeth spine-tipped. Corolla orange-brown. Nutlets obliquely truncate.

Flowering and fruiting: September-December

Distribution: Cultivated and naturalised throughout the hotter parts of India, from the Punjab to Travancore and Singapore, and in the regions of Ceylon.

Leonotis nepetaefolia R. Br.

Tall erect annual A-6 ft. high. Stem stout, puberulous, bluntly 4-angled deeply sulcate, the faces concave. Leaves membranous, about 2.5-6 in. long ovate, acute, coarsely crenate-serrate, puberulous on both sides, base cuneate; petioles 1-4 in. long, winged above. Whorls axillary, floral leaves lanceolate, deflexed; bracts deflexed, linear, hairy, spine-pointed. Calyx 3/4 in. long, ribbed, puberulous below, upper part densely villous and clothed with long white bristly hairs, tube incurved, mouth oblique, throat glabrous; teeth unequal, spine-tipped, the upper one up to 1/3 in. long, ovate, acute, the rest smaller and triangular. Corolla orange scarlet; tube 1/3 in. long, globrous below, upper part hairy, inside with 3 parallel rings of white hairs, upper part 1/4 in. long, densely woolly, lower 1/8-1/3 in. long. Nutlets 1/4 in. long, obliqually truncate, linear-oblong, widening upwards.

Plant cultivated and naturalised in most parts of the area within Upper Gangetic Plains and adjacent Siwalik and neighbouring region, but chiefly in the vicinity of villages.

It is found throughout the hotter parts of India and in the drier parts of Ceylon, widely spread also in South-east Asia. Tropical America and in Africa.

Leonotis nepetifolia (L.) R.Br. ('nepetaefolia'). Glabrous undershrubs. Blade ovate-lanceolate, up to 7X4 cm. membranous. Verticillasters 8 cm. across. Calyx tube hairy, 1.5 cm. long, bent above the middle; teeth 8, spinescent unequal, posterior tooth the longest. Corolla 2 cm. long, orange.

Tropical Asia, Africa and America. India; southern India, plant fairly common along hedges in plains, Karnataka.

Genus *Leonotis* R. Brown in the family Lamiaceae with salient features. Inflorescence a verticillasters Calyx tubular, 10-nerved; mouth oblique; teeth 8-10. Corolla 2-lipped; tube annulate within; upper lip erect, hooded, densely woolly at apex, entire; lower lip small, 4-lobed. Stamens didynamous, anterior pair the longest; filaments ascending under the upper lip, warted; anther cells divergent. Style very unequally bifid.

Genus *Leonotis* R. Br. (about 12 species mostly African, one of which occurs also in India and America; or 2 species naturalised and cultivated throughout, 40 tropical and South African species and 1 pantropical species) has specific characters of flower is with calyx 8 to 10-toothed and teeth spinescent that differs from genus *Roylea* Wall. by calyx 5-lobed, segments obovate-oblong, as both genera have calyx-lobes obovate-oblong, and upper lip of corolla hooded.

In a big family Lamiaceae or Labiatae, the genus *Leonotis* belongs to tribe 5 Stchydeae and subtribe 3 Lamieae comprising genera with common character of 5-toothed calyx, anther cells divergent and nutlets obtuse, and distinguishing character genus in particular as calyx 8-10-toothed and corolla lower lip very small. These genera come under a group with general characters of upper lip of corolla hooded and villous, and genus *Leonotis* is distinguishable. It is very striking-looking plant in flowering stage. Its lower lip of corolla longer than the upper lip, and it is separated from *Leucas* R. Br. by lower lip of corolla longer than the upper lip in its flower.

The root, leaves, flower-heads, seeds, stem and whole plant of *Leonotis nepetaefolia* R.Br. are medicinally useful.

The seeds possess feeble anti-malarial activity. The plant is considered useful in skin affcetions. Ashes of flowers are applied to scalds and burns. The whole plant is considered depurative, emmenagogue, febrifuge, laxative and narcotic, and used in skin diseases, amenorrohea and fevers.

Decoction of leaves is used as tonic and febrifuge. They are used in the treatment of rheumatic affections. Ashes of flower-heads mixed with curd or suitable media or vehicle considered useful for external application in ringworms and itchy affections.

Roots of the plant are crushed and rubbed on the breast when it swells and milk does not pass through the nipples. Decoction of leaves is useful as tonic.

The infusion of roots and leaves or juice of leaves may be useful as febrifuge in doses of 2 drachms to 2 ounces of infusion for oral intake in fever and as bitter tonic in general debility also.

Leaves are burnt and their ash is applied over burns. Flowers are useful as external application in eczema, cuts, wounds and sores. Ash of inflorescence finely is considered useful in eye complaints. Flowers calyx is useful in stomach pains. Stems are useful in bodyache and swelling on body.

Seeds are useful in wounds, malarial fever, febrile condition, dropsy, urinary troubles with lack of urine as diuretic.

Whole plant is useful in paralysis, convulsions, cramps and other ailments.

Leaves contain bitter substance. Seeds chemical analysis and screening of various parts find active constituents and other chemical components.

Seeds analysis finds the values moisture 8.8, either extract (fatty oil) 28.0, protein 23.6, crude fibre 14.3, N-free extr. 19.3 and ash 5.9%. Glucose, fruticose, and a phytin-like substance containing inositol, phophorous and calcium have been indentified. Steam-distillation or seeds yields 2 per cent of a volatile oil. The fatty oil extracted from seeds is similar to olive oil which has the particular characterstics including the saponin, iodine, acid, unsaponin matter, acetate and other values. The component fatty acids of the oil are linoleic 11.9, oleic 64.6, myristic 1.3, palmitic 12.0 and stearic 1.3 per cent.

Leaves yield a bitter principle, fatty oil (1%), resin, resinic acid and ash (7%), calyx and flowers contain these similar substance. Traces of an alkaloid-like compound are present in various parts of the plant, and the seeds possess feeble anti-malarial activity.

Leonotis leonurus R. Br., the plant grown in Indian gardens for ornament, is reported to possess medicinal efficacy. The leaves contain two phenolic compounds, a resin and a reddish oil with a high boiling point. The plant is mildly anthelmintic but too weak to be of practical value. It is also feebly narcotic. A decoction of leaves is used as purgative and as an emmenagogue in. Plant is also used for coughs and colds.

Medicinal properties and action of plant drug-Rasa tikta-kasāya, Vīrya uṣṇa, Guṇa laghu; Vatapitta sāmaka (tridoṣahara); Karma jvaraghna, kandughna, vraṇaropaṇa, sāraka, madakāri, dīpana, vadanāsthāpana, balya, tvacya, artavajanana, mutrala, ākṣepahara, kaṭupauṣṭika, angamarda-prasamana, nāḍībalya, and cakṣuṣya. Therapeutic indication in Jvara, viṣamajvara, dadru, kaṇḍū, vraṇa, kṣata, agnidagdha, jalodara, mūtravikāra, mūtrakṛccha, tvacāvikāra, daurbalya, pakṣāghāta, ākṣepa, pāmā-vicarcikā, āmāsayasūla, ārtavavikāra and vibandha, and other various ailments.

Kaṇṭapuṣpā, the Sanskrit name for plant drug.

10

Lepidagathis cristata Willd.

Family: Acanthaecae

Regional names: Kolichechutar (Bombay) Karappanpundu, (Malayalam) Bhuiterada, Bhuyaterada-(Marathi), Otdhompo (Santhal); Chilbethka

Perennial herb with procumbent branches. Leaves linear or oblong, up to 4.7x1 cm. Spikes aggregated at the base in globose, radical or subradical heads. Flowers white, spotted with brown and purple. Bracts and calyx lobes spinous-mucronate. Capsules 2-seeded.

Flowering and fruiing: October-April

Plant occurring commonly on the Ridge of Delhi in the shade of trees and rare in other places northern India. Southern India or occasional in other regions;

Lepidagathis cristata Willd.

Herb creeping from a stout rootstock. Leaves up to 2.5 x 0.8 cm., linear-oblong, glabrous. Spikes capitate, mostly crowded on lower nodes. Bracts pubescent, white-margined, spinescent. Clayx-lobes bract-like with a short spine. Corolla hairy, white; lower lip with middle lobe larger and pinkish. Anther cells unequally placed, hairy along dehiscing lines.

Distribution: Central and Eastern Peninsular India; Konkan, Deccan North Circars and Carnatic, and other regions.

Plant occurring as common herb in gravelly terrain in the eastern plains, Karnataka; Herb flowering in all seasons.

Lepidagathis hamiltoniana Wall.

(under *Lepidagathis cristata* var. *rupestris*)

Regional names: Gharia (Mundari); Bhuinium

Family: Acanthaceae

Perennial herb. Stems elongate, flageliform, leafy upwards. Leaves 5-6 in. long, linear or narrowly oblong, subfalcate, nearly glabrous, margins scabrous. Spikes in globular heads, arising from the base of the stems; bracts up to 1/2 in. long white spreading hairs. Calyx-segments membranous, tough, lanceolate, acuminate, spirescent, not thickened upwards, the lower one broader and bifid. Corolla strigose outside with white hairs, spotted with brown inside. Capsule 2-seeded, conical scarious on the back, thin and irregularly rupturing. Seeds ovate, covered with long hairs.

Distribution: Bihar, Chota Nagpur and southwards in Chanda in the Central Provinces.

Plant occurring in dry situations and in the Jamuna ravines, Brijabhumi and adjacent parts, Bundelkhand; Madhya Bharata, Rajputana, North Oudha; Central India, U.P., M.P., Bihar, Upper Gangetic Plains and other regions.

Lepidagathis incurva D.Don. var. **mucronata** (Nees.) C.B. Clarke

Lepidagathis mucronata Nees.

L. hyalina var. *mucronata* (Hees.) C.B. Clarke

Family: Acathaceae

Erect herbs. Leaves 5-10 x 2-3.5 cm. obovate, long-tapered to petiole, pubescent, beneath. Spikes capitate and axillary.

Bracts ovate-acute, spinescent, pilose-hairy. Calyx lobes bract-like. Corolla white pink dots on lower lip, hairy without, less than 1 cm. long.

Flowering and fruiting: December-March.

Distribution: South Western India. Plant common in Ghats, along edges of wet deciduous or semi-evergreen forests, in forests clearings and cardamon estates.

Lepidagathis trinervis Nees.

Family: Acanthaceae

Regional names: Harancharo, Paniru (Gujarati)

Diffuse perennial herb, woody below; branches many, 5-10 in. long, slender, 4-angled. Leaves sessile, 1-1.4 in. long, linear, subàcute, entire, nearly glabrous, 3-nerved from a tapering base, margins scabrous. Flowers in axillary, ovoid spikes 1/2-3//4 in. long, usually 2 or more spikes, closely packed together and forming that appears to be single head; bracts under 1/2 in. long, ovate or obovate, tipped with a long recurved spine; bracteoles as long as bracts, oblong lanceolate, aristate, softly membranous. Calyx membranous, 3 outer segments, nearly equal in length, lanceolate, acute-spine-pointed, nearly glabrous outside, very hairy within; the 2 inner lateral segments shorter and narrower, hairy on both sides. Corolla white with yellow brown or purple spots 1/4-1/3 in long. Capsule 2-seeded, 1/4 in. long, ovoid-lanceolate, subacute, with and bursting irregularly. Seeds covered with long hairs.

Flowering and fruiting: Cold season and onwards.

Distribution: North-West Himalayas, Chota Nagpur and at the base of Sikkim hills, extending to Central Western and Southern India.

Plant frequently occurring in Merwara (Rajsthan) in dry rocky or sandy ground.

Lepidagathis incurva Buch-Ham ex D. Don.

Lepidagathis hyalina Nees.
L. incurva D.Don.

Ruellia dependens Roxb.
Family: Acanthaceae
Regional names: Charemomorkha

Suberect perennial herb, 1-2 ft. high, or the stems often somewhat prostrate. Leaves about 3 in. long, minutely glandular-hairy, scabrous on the nerves beneath; lower ovate; upper narrower, pendent, petioles 1/2 in. long. Spike oblong, dense, axillary and terminal, often clustered, softly hairy; bracts nearly 1/2 in. long, lanceolate, acuminate, mucronate; bracteoles 1/3 in. long narrower. Calyx 1/3 in. long, linear-lanceolate, mucronate, outer segments longest. Corolla 1/4 in. long, white with brown spots on the palate.

Flowering and fruiting: Autumn to Summers

Distribution: Outer Himalayan ranges from the Punjab eastwards, up to 4,000 in Kumaon; also in Bengal, North Assam and Burma, extending to China.

Plant abundantly occurring within the areas of Upper Gangetic Plains, and especially in the Sub-Himalayan tracts.

Lepidagathis incurva Buch.-Ham. ex D.Don. syn. *Lepidagathis hyalina* Nees.

Perennial herb. Leaves petioled ovate or oblong, minutely viscid pubescent, uppermost often narrower, pendent, undulate. Spikes oblong, very dense, axillary and terminal, often clustered, ciliate, often softly hairy, erect, 1-seeded; bract lanceolate, acuminate mucronate. Calyx sub-partite, segments linear-lanceolate, mucronate, outer larger, sometimes softly hairy. Corolla white with brown spotted palate. Capsule 4-seeded.

Throughout India from Jammu to Upper Assam. Plant occurring in the foot hills of Kumaon region, ascending to 1500 m. elevation. Herb flowering in March-April, and fruiting in April-May.

Leidagathis incurva Buch.-Ham. ex D.Don. Erect or decumbent-ascending or clambering, perennial herbs, with a woody base. Stems often much-branched from the base, pubescent towards the apex. Leaves subequal, ovate-lanceolate, rounded, often decurrent at base, acute or acuminate, serrate-dentate, hairy. Petiole 0.5-2 cm. long. Bracts glandular-hairy in the upper parts, 0.7-1 cm. long. Bracteoles 0.8 cm. long. Calyx 0.9-1 cm. long, villous on the back; segments lanceolate, acuminate. Corolla white, 1-1.2 cm. long, with a brown-spotted, villous throat. Capsule short hairy, 0.6-0.65 cm. long.

Plant commonly occurring in sal forestes, forests edges and scrub jungles; Siwaliks, Uttar Pradesh. Herb flowering during November to May.

Lepidagathis cuspidata Nees.

Family: Acathaceae

Erect undershrub. Stems 1-3 ft. high; branches 4-angled, often gland-pubescent upwards. Leaves of main stem 3—3.5 in. long, oblong-lanceolate, acute or acuminate, usually mucronate, glabrous or nearly so, tapering of the base and decurrent into the petiole; leaves of the branches subsessile and much smaller, elliptilic-lanceolate, spinous, pointed, softly hairy. Spikes terminal or terminating shrot axillary branches, varying in length according as the flower densely or loosely arranged, and if the later, the flowers distinctly in opposite pairs; bracts about 1/2 in. long, elliptic or obovate, acute, spine-tipped, 3-5nerve gland-hairy; outer segments longer, broader than the inner, spine-tipped; the 2 inner lateral segments linear acute. Corolla white streaked with purple; upper lip oval, acute; lower lip with rounded lobes, palate glabrous. Seeds clothed with short hairs especially along the margins.

Flowering and fruiting:	March-May; January-June
Distribution:	Western Himalayas, localities up to 5,000 ft. alt., in Kumaon, extending to Central and Western India.

Lepidagathis cuspidata Nees.

Erect suffruticose, perennial herbs or undershrubs. Stems often decumbent, ascending, narrowly margined, glandular hairy towards the apex. Leaves subsessile or on short petioles, in unequal pairs, obovate-spatulate, narrowed to the base, acuminate or acute, mucronate; those on branchlets smaller, ovate-elliptic, rounded at base, cuspidate with an apicular tip, glandular, pubescent. Flowers in subsessile or short-peduncled, 3-10 cm. long spikes. Bracts ciliate, 0.5-1 cm. broad. Bracteoles lanceolate, spine-tipped, 0.8 cm. long. Clayx 1-1.2 cm. long; segments unequal, lanceolate, gland-ciliate, hairy on the back. Corolla white, 1.4-1.5 cm. long. Capsule glabrous, 0.9-1 cm. long.

Plant commonly occurring roadsides, waste places, forest edges, forest clearings scrub jungles and sal forests; Siwalik range, Upper Gangetic Plains, and along the sub-Himalayan tracts eastwards to eastern Uttar Pradesh region bordering Nepal, and Terai of Nepal. Herb flowering during the period from spring to summer.

Lepidagathis cuspidata Nees.

Erect shrub. Leaves elliptic at both ends, puberulous, petiole small. Leaves on the lateral flowering branches small, mucronate. Spike dense or lax with flowers in distinct opposite pairs; bracts ovate, cuspidate, 3-nerved. Corolla whitish with purple spots. Capsule 4-seeded.

Plant occurring common on steep bare rocky or shady slopes, on road cuttings and similar exposed situations; Kumaon region, ascending to 1500 m. elevation, in sub-Himalayan tract and outer Himalayas from Ravi eastwards. Plant flowering in February to April, and fruiting in April to May or onwards as these stages begin during winters and end by summers generally, as the flowering commences when all the leaves have fallen from the plants mostly.

Lepidagathis purpuricaulis Nees.

Family: Acanthaceae

Erect or decumbent-ascending or clambering perennial herbs, with a woody base. Stems often branched from the base, 4-gonous, often purple-tinged. Leaves unequal, oblanceolate-obovate, narrowed towards the base, acute or acuminate, glabrous, 2-10 x 0.5-3 cm. Flowers in crowded spikes. Bracts lanceolate, glandular hairy, 0.6-0.7 cm. long. Bracteoles 0.8-1 cm. long. Calyx-segments very unequal, linear-lanceolate, gland-ciliate, 0.7-1 cm. long. Corolla pale purple, 1-1.5 cm. long.

Flowering and fruiting: March-June

Distribution: Sub-Tropical Western Himalayas up to 4,000 ft. elevation in Kumaon region, Chota Nagpur, extending to Burma.

Plant commonly occurring in sal forests, forest edges and scrub jungles; Siwalik range, foot hills, Uttar Pradesh. Some other species of *Lepidagathis* Willd. in relevançe may be indicated:-

Lepidagathis incurva var. *mollis* (Cl.) Raizadas Saxena

L. hyalina Neels. var. *mollis* Cl.

Lipidagathis incurva var. *mucronata* (Nees.) Cl.

L. mucronata Nees.

L. hyalina var. *mucronata* (Nees.) Cl.

Lepidagathis incurva var. *astulata* (Nees) R. & S.

L. astulata Nees.

L. hyalina var. *astulata* (Nees.) Cl.

Genus *Lepidagathis* Willd. in the family Acanthaceae (about 250 genera and chiefly 2,500 species; and about 68 genera with over 337 species in India) has about 100 tropical and subtropical species which include about 28 species in India, mostly in Southern and Western India.

Salient features of genus *Lepidagathis* Willd.-Herbs or under shrubs, with often pubescent bracts or leaves. Leaves entire or crenate serrate. Flowers sessile, usually capitate, sometime opposite or soliatary; head terminal or axillary, dense, usually 1-seeded, often fascicled; bracts usually larger than the calyx segments, rarely small; bracteoles narrower than the bracts. Calyx deeply 5-lobed; segments unequal, the 2 anterior more or less connate (calyx 4-partite) corolla small, tubular, suddenly ventricose in the middle, didynamous; anthers all 2-celled, cells oblong, muticus, parallel or one lower somewhat divergent. Stigma capitellate, minutely bifid or entire. Capsule 2 or 4-seeded, elongate, conoid or oblong. Seeds compressed, hairy.

Relevant species of the genus *Lepidagathis* Willd. may be distinguished on the basis of various characters.

Lepdagathis incurva Buch-Ham ex D.Don is a perennial herb, with leaves minutely, viscid-pubescent, and flowers white with brown spots. Comparatively *Lepidagathis cuspidata* Nees. is shrubby plant, with leaves puberulous at both ends, and flowers whitish with purplish spots. Spikes clustered at base of stems in *Lepidagathis cristata* Willd., but spikes not clustered at base of stems in *Lepidagathis incurva* var. *mucronata* (Nees.) C.B. Clarke.

Genus *Lepidagathis* Willd. is specific of plants with erect or; prostrate, with stems and cauline leaves, and particularly spikes aggregated in radical or subradical globose heads. Flower with 3-lobed calyx, 4 stamens, and bracts and bracteoles similar, ending in spinescent pungent tips. All stamens perfect included, and corolla less than 2 cm. long (corolla-segments imbricate in buds.)

Important species of genus *Lepidagathis* Willdenow differ for floral characterstics. *Lepidagathis cuspidata* Nees. has ovate-elliptic bracts with an apiculate-tipped top, penni-nerved, and with spikes solitary, cylindric, not secund; whereas lanceolate, acuminate bracts with an apical mucro, parallel-nerved, and spikes in clusters, secund in other some species which are further distinguishable on the basis of specific flower characters. *Lepidagathis purpuricaulis* Nees. has bracts with 0.03-0.08 cm. long cilia, marginal nerves prominent, spikes hairy or pubescent, and corolla pale puple; whereas bracts with ± 0.2 cm. long cilia, marginal nerves faint, spikes softly villous and corolla white in *Lepidagathis incurva* Buch-Ham ex D.Don.

Species with common characters of capsules 2-seeded, bursting irregularly and seeds clothed with long hairs are separated of characterstic calyx such as calyx-lobes are spinescent in *Lepidagathis hamiltoniana* Wall., when calyx-lobes are not spinescent in *Lepidagathis trinervis* Nees. Similarly the species with 4-seeded capsules, distinctly 2-valved and seeds clothed with short hairs, are primarily separable of their plants habit and further distinguishable for lower characters. For the instance, *Lepidagathis cuspidata* Nees. erect undershrub are with bracts and calyx-segments glandular-hairy; whereas the diffuse or prostrate herbs, rarely suberect, of a few species, differ for characterstic bracts, such as bracts striate in *Lepidagathis purpuricaulis* Nees. when bracts not striate in *Lepidagathis hyalina* Nees.

In general, a few species like *Lepidagathis incurva* Buch-Ham ex D.Don. and *L. purpuricaulis* Nees. are variable in habit, hairiness, shape of leaves, size and length of spikes. The leaves, roots, flowers, seeds and whole plant of various species of *Lepidagathis* Willd. are medicinally useful.

Lepidagathis cristata Willd. is bitter herb which is useful as tonic in fever. Herb is applied to cure itchy affections of skin. Ash of drug plant is used as application to sores. Whole plant is burnt to prepare the ash which is then externally applied over the sores, and the same is also useful for applying in skin affections like itch, scabies and similar complaints. The plant decoction or powder is given in fever as bitter tonic.

Whole plant is considered an antiallergic medicine and it is used in various allergic affections particularly or skins and dermatological complaints.

Herb is useful in scabies, boils, sores, syphilis, wounds and boils of head. External application is generally made. Whole plant paste is applied for its haemostatic utility over fresh cuts and other conditions.

Plant is febrifuge and given in the forms of infusion or decoction in fevers, and general debility during febrile conditions in patients.

The leaves of the plant are also used as fodder. Leaves contain (values on dry basis) protein 9.25, fat (ether ext.) 3.90, carbohydrates 40.85, fibres 32.56; ash 13.44, iron 1.32, calcium 1.97, phophorous 0.31, and silica 6.24 per cent.

The roots of plant *Lepidagathis hamiltoniana* Wall. are crushed and rubbed on breast when swollen and milk does not pass through the nipples or less of lactation due to mammary swelling.

The whorl in flower or in seed is pounded and fried in Karanj oil rubbed on itch, also on head sores in children. Whole plant is useful in skin affections as external applications.

Leaves of the plant are useful for applying to itchy complaints of skin and sores.

The roots of herb are particularly considered stomachic and useful in dyspepsia and other conditions.

The fruit, leaves and whole plant of *Lepidagathis incurva* D.Don. syn. *L. hyalina* Nees. are medicinally useful.

The leaves of the plant are considered useful against cough, and for this purpose the leaves when chewed to help relief from cough and similar cough ailments. The fruits are considered useful in ear complaints.

Whole plant of *Lepidagathis trinervis* Nees. are medicinal useful and other parts are also considered medicinal.

Decoction or infusion of whole plant is given as bitter tonic and specially useful in fevers.

Medicinal properties and actions of the plant drug-Rasa Tikta-kasāya, Virya uṣṇa, Vipaka kaṭu, Guṇa laghu; Karma balya, katupauṣṭika, jvaraghna, vraṇaropaṇa, kaṇḍughna, tvacya, Sothahara, vedanāsthāpana, dīpana, raktarodhaka and kasahara; and therapeutic indication in various diseases such as Jvara, kasa, phiraṅga, tvacaroga, kaṇḍū, vraṇa, siro-vraṇa, kṣata, anurjata, vraṇasotha, stanasotha, karṇaroga and daurbalya.

Sūryakaṇṭhā, Sṛgālapadī and Chillatiṣṭhā, the Sanskrit names for the plant drug.

Section - III

1

Atylosia scarabaeoides (Linn.) Benth.

Dolichos scarabaeoides Linn.

Cantharospermum pauciflorum Wright & Arnot.

Family: Fabaceae (Papilicanaceae)

Regional names: Karbani, Birghore, Bankulthi; Walhollu

Silender, twining or trailing, often suberect at first, hairy pubescent, annual-perennial herbs. leaflets elliptic -obvoate, to oblong, obtuse or rounded and mucronate at apex, rounded at base, plubescent, gland-dotted beneath; terminal leaflets on 0.5-0.7 cm. long petiolulues; lateral ones subsessile. Petiole 1.5-4(-5) cm. long. Flowers 0.8-1 cm. long, corymbose-racemes or often reduced to 1-2 on short peduncles. Bracts small, 0.1-0.15 cm. long. Calyx 0.7-0.75 cm, long. Corolla slightly exerted; standard 0.8-0.9 (-1) cm. long. Style 0.6 cm. long. Pod 2 to 6-seeded, densely clothed with appressed-haris. Seeds 0.4-0.5 X 0.3 cm.

Flowering and fruiting : August - December

Distribution : Throughout India, ascending to 5,000 ft. on the Western Himalyas. Also in Malaya, China, Mauritius and Madagascar.

Atylosia scarabaeoides Benth.

Slender herbaceous twiner with densely grey-downy stems. Leaves 1 to 2 in. long, subdigitately 3-foliolate; stipules minute, cadacous. Leauflets obovate-oblong, obtuse or subacute, subcoriaceous, 3-nerved towards the base thinly grey-canescent above, pubescent and faintly reticulate-veined beneath, petioled. Racemes 2-6-flowered, on densely pubescent short axillary peduncles; Calyx densely grey-silky, teeth linear, the lowest twice as long as the tube. Corollas yellow, keel abruptly incurved at the tip. Pods straight 3/4 -1 in. long, 4-6 seeded, clothed with fine spreading brown silky hairs, the transverse lines slightly oblique.

Plant occurring commonly within the area of Upper Gangetic Plains and adjacent regions.

Atylosia scasrabaeoides (Linn.) Benth. A. slender, twining or trailing herb common in grassy areas, roadsides, waysides, forest clearing and scrub jungles, Siwaliks and sub-Himalayan tracts; , and the plains in northern India.

From Hosiarpur eastwards. Plant flowering most of the year. Flowers yellow, in axillary clusters of 2-6 and petals soon falling off.

Atylosia volubilis (Blance) Gamble

Cytisus velubilis Blance

Atylesia mollis sensu Baker

A. orassa Prain.

Cantharospermum volubile (Blance) Merr.

Family : Fabaceae

Regional names : Bajhala

Stout climbers or twiners. Branches, particularly young ones, densely patently short-hairy with brownish hairs. Leaflets acuminate at apex; terminal one on 0.4-0.5 cm. long petiolules, rhomboid, cuneate at base; lateral ones ovate - elliptic, 0.2-0.25 cm. long petiolules, subtruncate at base, glabrate or finely hairy above, densely softly pubescent, with numerous yellow or organe-coloured dots on the lower surface. Petiole 3-3.5 (-4) cm. long. Stipules 0.33 cm. long, persistent. Flowers yellow, 1.8.2 cm. long, in short-hairy racemes or in panicles of 2-8 (-10) cm. long (incl. 0.5-4 cm. long peduncle). Bracts acute, densely short-hairy on the back, 1.5-1.8 (-2) X 0.7-0.8 cm., caducous. Pedicels 0.5-0.7 cm. long. Calyx 0.7-0.8 (-1) cm. long, glandular-viscid-hairy; lobes ovate-triangular, acute, upper two connate up to the apex; standard retuse. Style hairy in the upper half. Pod densely patently short-hairy, glandular-punctate, 2.3-5 X 1-1.5 cm. to 6-seeded.

Flowing and fruiting : January - May
Distribution:

Atylosia mollis Benth.

(excl. all syns. except *Callaces mollis*)
Family : Fabaceaue

Densely pubescent herb. Stemp twining, long. Leaflets ovate, longer than broad, coriaceous, shortly papillose above, persistently grey down beneath. Flowers short peduncled in raceme, yellow; bracteolas large, roundish, forming a conspicuous tuft before the racemes expand. Petals yellow, twice the length of calyx. Pods straight grey pubescent, 8-10 seeded..

Flowering and Fruiting : September - October

Distribution : In Sub-Himalayan tract from Rawalpindi to Sikkim (600-2000 metres; from Chamba to North-West Himalaya to eastern Himalayan parts, Sikkim.

Atylosis mollis Benth. A twining herb with firm slender glabrascent branches. Leaves beneath densely and uniformally grey-downy, not reticulate. Leaflets much longer than broad. Flowers yellow, over 1 in, long. Pod 2 in.

transverse depressons between the seeds at right angles to the sutures. Seeds 8-10, their longer diameter scross the pod.

Plant occurring in Siwalik range and sub-Himalayan tracts.

Atylosia platycarpa Benth.

Family : Fabaceia

Slender, trailing or twtining hirsute-hairy, annual herbs. Leaflets broadly ovate-elliptic, abruptly acuminate at apex, glandular-punctate beneath, hairy. Petiole 6-8 (-10) cm. long. Flowers 1-2, on 2-2.5 cm. long peduncles. Pedicels 1.2-1.5 cm. long. Bracts ovate, acuminate, 0.4-0.5 cm. long. Calyx 1.3-1.5 cm. long, hirsute on the back; segments ovate-lanceolate, acuminate. Standard truncate at apex. Pod 5 to 7- seeded, clothed with patent, deciduous hairs. Seeds ovoid, black.

Flowering and fruiting : August - November

Distribution : Bengal, Central Provinces, Uttar Pradesh, Madhya Pradesh, and up to 8,000 ft. on Western Himalayas.

Atylosia platycarpa Benth. A twining or trailing herb with very slender grey-pubescent branches. Leaves 3-foliolate; leaflets 1-3 in. long, the terminal one distinctly stalked, roundish, acute or acuminate-cuspidate, membranous, finely pilose on both surfaces; peduncles shorter than the petioles, suppressed at the ends of the shoots, where the leaves also are much reduced, 1-2-flowered; pedicels as long as the calyx, Calyx densely pilose, teeth linear-setaceous. Corolla little exerted. Pod 1-1 3/4 in. long, straight, flat, distinctly lineate thinly pilose, 5-7 seeded.

Plant occurring in Swillik range, Upper Gangetic plans, Uttar Pradesh, Madhya Pradesh, Central India. Common herb in grassy fields, roadsides and agricultural fields.

Atylosia lineata Wight. & Arnot.

Atylosis lawii Wight.

Family : Fabaceae

Regional names : Rantur

Softly hirsute, erect undershurbs, Leaflets subacute, up to 4 x 1.5 cm., membranous, pulsecent beneath.

Flowers pairs on minute peduncle, 1.4 cm. long. Calyx teeth equalling the tube. Corolla yellow, marcescent. Pod grey-silky-pubescent, 2 X 0.6 cm. 2-3-seeded.

Flowering and fruiting : All seasons

Distribution : South-West India. Frequent in wet deciduous forests, Karnataka.

Atylosia albicans (Wight. & Ar.) Bentham

Cantharospermum albicaus Wight. & Arn.

Family : Fabaceae

Grey-canescent climbing shrubs. Leaflets obtuse, up to 3 X 2.7 cm. densely pubescent beneath, chartaceuous. Raceme slender, 3-5 cm. long, few-flowered. Calyx teeth shorter than tube. Corolla yellow, 2 cm. long. Pod white-pubescent, 4 X 1 cm., 5-7 seeded.

Flowering and fruiting : September - November

Distribution : South-West India, Sri Lanka, Occasional in scrub, Karnataka.

Atylosia elongata Benth.

Herbaceous twiner, clothed with fine, spreading hairs, Leaflets 3, narrowed from the middle to a rounded base, pointed. Flowers long-peduncled. Pods oblong.

Plant occasional in Delhi area; Northern India, Nepal Khasia and Assam. Herb flowering in August-September.

Atylosia goensis (Dalz.) Linn.

Cajanus goensis Dalz.

Dunbaria barbata Benth.

Attylosia barbata (Benth.) Baker

Family : Fabaceae

Woody climber; branches densely pubescent, leaftlets roundish stipellate subcordiaceous thinly shortly pubescent, Branches firm, densely clothed at first with short spreading grey pubescence. Stipules short, lanceolatte, caducous; petiole 1-4 in. long; leaflets 3-4 in. broad and long, cuspidate, broadly rounded at the base, green above., paler and greyer beneath, both surfaces minutely permanently pubescent; peduncles often overtopping the leaves; racemes at firstclose finally 4-6 in. long, the rachis densely pilose; bracts roundish or ovate, with a cusp. shaggy, exceeding the buds. Calyx shaggy, teeth lanceolate, exceeding the tube. Standard half as long again as the calyx, keel equalling the calyx 1/2 in. bread. Flowers in long-peduncled recemes. Pods short, straight, densely clothed with long grey spreading hairs, narrowed to both ends; pods 5 - seeded.

Distribution : Assam, Tenasserim, Concan. Java.

Genus *Atylosia* Wright. & Arnott. in family Fabaceae or Papilionaceae, sub-family of Leguminoseae, with salient features- Herbs or shrubs, erect or twining. Leaves 3 - foliolate, sometimes subdigitate, often exstipellate. gland-dotted beneath. Flowers axillary or racemed. Calyx-teeth distinct, longer or shorter than the tube, tthe lowest the longest. Corolla more or less exerted, merascent or canducous; keel not beaked. Stamens 2-adalphous, anthers uniform. Ovary sessile; style filiform, incurved, glabrous; stigma capitate; ovules 3. Pod linear or oblong, turgid, marked with transverse lines between the seeds which have a conspicuous divided strophiole.

Genus *Atylosia* Wt. & Arn. in family Fabaceae (Papilionaceae, the largest of the three suborders of Leguminoseae, a very large order of Dicot class) has about 25 species from India to Australia and Mauritius. In distributional pattern, the species of genus *Atylosia* W. & A. spread that twentyone species in tropical Asia and Australia one in tropical Africa and Madagascar; shrubs or herbs, erect or climbing; sixteen species in India, mostly in Western Peninsular India, a few in tropical and subtropical Himalayas.

Genus *Atylosia* W. & A. belongs to tribue III Phaseoleae (sub-tribe Cajaneae - leaves gland-dotted beneath) and a group of genera having ovules 3 to many; and the characters of pods with depressed lines between the seeds in two genera namely *Atylosia.* W. & A. and *Cajanus* DC. which may be separated by character of seeds as the seeds of *Atylosia* are strophiolate. Genera with pods more than 2-seeded have a common character that valves of pod with oblique, deep depressions between the seeds; and the seeds carunculate in twiner plants of *Atylosia* W. & A. when the same become ecarunculate in erect plants of latter genera (*Cajanus* DC.). Though various genera plants have commonly leaves disitately or pinnately 1 to 3 - foliolate; and two genera *Maughania* ___ St.-Hill. and *Rhynchosia* Lour. may be separated from *Atylosia* W. & A. by 1 to 2-seeded pods in these genera when *Atylosis* pods are with more than 2 seeds besides other specific characters.

In general three genera of subtribe Cajaninae are with gland-dotted leaves beneath, leaflets exstipellatte and beardless style, and these are further distinguished of pods, number of seeds and other characters. Pods of *Atylosia* W. & A. have 3 or more seeds which are arillate.

Various species of genus *Atylosia* Wt. & Ant. are distinguishable by specific characters mainly of leaves, pods, stems and flowers, besides other morphological features.

Leaves stipellate; bracts boat-shaped, 1.5-1.7 X 0.7-0.8 cm.; flowers 1.5-2 (-2.3) cm. long; corolla persistent till maturity of the pod and stems climbers or twiners commonly in the two species *Atylosia volubilis* (Blanco) Gamble and *Atylosia mollis* Bentham, which are separated by number of seeds in their pods as pods 3 to 6-seeded in former species and 8 to 10 - seeded in the latter species.

Atylosis platycarpa Bentham and *Atylosia scarabaeoides* (Linn.) Bentham are both slender twiners with leaves exstipellate; bracts upto 0.5 cm. long; flowers 0.8-1.5 cm. long and corolla caducous; but these two species are distinguishable by other characters of stems, pods and leaflets.

Stems clothed with long, patent, ferruginous hairs of 0.25-6.3 cm. long and small, greyish brown hairs; leaflets 3.5-1.5 cm. reticulate-venose in *Atylosia, platycarpa*; whereas stems devoid of long, patent, ferruginous hairs; leaflets 2-3 X 1.1.5 cm. and pod -0.5-0.6 cm. mooth or faintly reticulate in *Atylosia scarabaeoides.*

Two species in South-West Indian regions differ each other for stem habit, leaflets and flowers characters. *Atylosia albicans* (Wight. & Arn.) Bentham plants are climbing with leaflets nearly as long as broad and flowers in racemes; whereas the plants erect with leaflets more than twice as long as broad and flowers in pairs in *Atylosia lineata* Wight. & Arn.

The species of genus *Atylosia* W. & A. may also be grouped for distinguishing them on the basis of flower characterstics. Broadly the petals marcescent in *Atylosia mollia* Bentham and *Atylesia crassa* Prin; whereas the petals falling before the pods develop in *Atylosia apicana* Benth., *Atylosia scarabaeoides* Benth. and *Attylosia platycarpa* Beath. These species differ in particular.

Firstly leaves not reticulate beneath and leaflets longer than broad in *Atylosia mollis;* when leaves strongly reticulate beneath and leaflet not longer than broad in *A. crass.*

Secondly, calyx-teeth short and corolla much exserted in. *Atylosia albican*; calyx teeth long and corolla little exserted in *A. scarabaeoides,* and both species have leaflets subdigitate. Terminal leaflet with an elongated stalk in *A. platycarpa.*

Vasrious species of *Atylosia* W. & A. are medicinally useful.

The roots of *Atylosia goensis* Dalz. are useful in rheumatism, biliousness, fever, consumption and swelling.

The roots *Atylosia volubilis Gamble.* are ground and made into a paste which is applied locally in mumps ailment.

Whole plant of *Atylosia mollis* Benth. and some other parts are medicinally used. Plant is useful in dropsy, anasarca, pain in lower limbs or legs and also for swelling during pregnancy.

The seeds of *Atylosia platycarpa* Benth. are useful in the eyes ailing with sores.

The leaves, roots, seeds and whole plant of *Atylosia scarabaeoides* Benth. are medicinally useful.

Leasves are useful in pre and post-natal care in females as they are used in child birth, swelling after pregnancy and other complaints during pregnancy and after child birth.

Leaves are useful in treating symphilis, gonorrhoea and other veneral diseases.

Leaves are given in treatment of some gastro-intestinal ailments. Leaves are used in cholera, dysentery, diarrhoea and gastric troubles.

Leaves are externally applied to wounds, sores and swelling caused with trauma, and also in bruises.

Leaves are considered useful for giving in cases of female sterility.

Whole plant is useful in gastric troubles, gonorrhoea, night fever and pain in legs. Whole plant is externally useful in bald and ailments of head.

Plant is useful in small pox, snake bite, veneral diseases, and other similar complaints. It is also used in anasarca.

Plant is externally applied to burns, sores and wounds.

Whole plant is useful in spermatorrhoea.

The seeds are edible.

In veterinary medicine, the whole plant to also useful in certain ailments of cattles.

Medicinal properties and action of plant drug - Rasa kaṭutikta, Vīrya uṣṇa. (nātyuṣṇasīta), Vipāka katu, Guna laghu; Vātapittahara (tyridoṣasamaka); and Karma vraṇaropaṇa, keṣya, vedanā-sthāpana, viṣaghna, dīpana, pācana, surajanana, saṅgrāhi, āmapācana, sūlaprasamana, sothahana, jvaraghna, raktasodhaka, prajāsthāpana, bandhyattvanāsana and nāḍībalya.

Therapeuic indication for internal and external uses in Jvasrs, visūcikā, rātrisveda -jvara, atisara, pravahika, kesaroga-indralupta, āmāsaya-āntra vikāra, jalodara, sotha, vrana, agnidaghda, ksata, sakthisūla, ratijaroga, upadaṁsa, phiranga, masurika, sukrameha, vīryavikāra, sarpaviṣa, garbhavyāpada, bandhyatva, garbhiṇīsetha, prasavottara vikāra, sotha, netraroga-vraṇa and other ailments.

Khādya - bīja

Pasucikitsā - pasuvikāra, pañcāṅga

Parṇakavallī, Sanskrit name for plant drug.

Bidens biternata (Lour.) Merr. & Sherff.

Corepsis biternata Lour.

Bidens pilosa auct. (non Linn.)

Family : Asteraceae (Compositae)

Regional names : Chirchita, Sui ka ped

Erect herb, 30-100 cm., tall. Leaves variable, simple or compound glabrous. Heads white or yellow, corymbosely panicled, heterogamous. Achenes 8-13 X 1 mm., quadrangular, ribbed, glabrous, black, Pappus 2-awned.

Flowering and fruiting : March-November

Plant occurring commonly in moist, shady places of gardens and long the banks of small channels of Delhi Canals and in various parts of Delhi area and adjoining Haryana, Punjab and Uttar Pradesh areas.

Bidens bipinnata Linn.

Bidens decomposita Wall ex DC

B. pilosa var. *bipinnata* (Linn.) Hook. f.

B. pilosa var. *ecomposita* (Wall ex DC) Hook.f.

Family : Asteraceae

Regional name :

Erect, simple or much-branched, annual herbs, up to 15-150 cm. tall. Stems 4-gonous, glabrous. Leaves oppositte, rarely upper ones alternate, 2 to 3 - pinnatipartite or pinnate, 4-20 cm. long; segments ovate-lanceolate, acute or acuminate, incised-serrate to lobulate, thinly hairy. Heads yellow, on ebracteate, 1-8 cm. long peduncles, 0.6-0 cm. across. Outer involcural bracts linear-spatulate, 0.25-0.26 (-0.3) cm. long; inner ones ovate-lanceolate, obttuse, 0.3-0.35 cm. long. Marginal flowers 2-4, with 2-globed corollas. Disk-flowers 0.3 cm. long. Achenes 4-angular, tapering towards the apex, glabrous or shortly hispid, 0.6-2 cm. long. Pappus setae 2-4, retrorsely bristly 0.25-0.3 cm. long.

Flowering and fruiting : March-November

Distribution : Throughout India

Bidens biternatea (Lour.) Merr. - Sherf. (= *Bidens pilosa* under *pilosa* proper sensu Hook. f.)

Erect herb. system rubust., glabrous near the base, pubescent upwards. Leaves oppoiste, 1-pinnate; leaflets 3-5 ovate, toothed. Heads radiate on long thick, diverging stalks; ligules white. Flower yellow or white; pappus of usually 3-bristles. Achenes linear, rough.

Distribution : Through India

Flowers and fruiting : August - October

Bidens wallichii Dc (= *Bidens pilosa* var. *bipinnata* sensu Hook. f.)

Erect herb. Stem robust. Leaves opposite, stalked, 2-pinnate, segments variously cut and lobed. Heads radiate on slender, diverging stalks. Flowers yellow or white; ligules yellow; pappus of usually 3- bristles. Achenes rough, linear.

Flowering and fruiting : August-September

Distribution : Throughout India

Bidens pilosa Linn.

Bidens bipinnata Linn.

Erect, glabrous or pubescent annual, 1-3 ft. high. Stems 4-angular, grooved, thickened at the neods. Leaves very variable, 3-fid, 3 foliolate or 1-2 pinnatifid; the terminal segments ovate, serratte; petioled dilated and sheathing at the base. Heads (in flower) about 1/2 in diam., elongating in fruit. Outer invol-bracts linear, obtuse, ciliate, shorter than the acute, broadly margined inner ones. Ray-flowers, lingulate, white or yellow. Ripe achenes small, slender, 4-angular, glabrous, black, exceeding the involucre. Pappus-awns spreading, yellow.

Flowering and fruiting : Rainy season to Autumn.

Distribution : Throughout India, ascending to 6,000 ft. in the Himalayas. Afaghanistan and in all warm countries.

Plant occurring commonly within the areas in Upper Gangetic Plains and adjacent regions.

Bidens pilosa Linn. (*quoad* var. *pilosa* ; excl. var.s *bipinnata* Hook. f. and *decomposita* Hook. f.

Erect simple or much-branched, annual herbs, up to 15-200 cm. tall Stems usually wide-branched, 4-gonous, striate, hairy. Leaves opposite, biternate or imparipinanate, usually 2 to 3-jugate; upper ones often simple; leaflets ovate-lanceolate to oblong, acute or acuminate, with a cuneate, shortly decurrent base, entire-serrate, glabrous or hairy on the nerves beneath, especially at the base, 4-10 X 1.8-5 cm. Heads 1. 2-1.5 cm. across, on 1-10 cm. long, hairy peduncles. Involucres campanulate; outer involucral bracts spatulate, acutely mucronate, nearly glabrous, not distinctly ciliate, 0.65-0.7 X 0.25 cm. ; inner ones lanceolate-oblong, obtuse, 0.5-1.5 cm. long. Marginal flowers 4-5, with white, 3- denate, 0.5-0.6 cm., long ligules. Disk-flowers with 0.4 cm., with 0.4 cm. long corollas. Achenes 0.7-1 cm. long, glabrous except hispid, narrowed top. Pappus-setae 2-4, retrorsely bristly, 0.12-0.3 cm. long.

Flowering and fruiting : March - November

Distribution : Throughout India

Plant occurring commonly in garden, roadsides, waste places, agricultural fields, orchards, river-beds and other places; Siwaliks and adjacent plains.

Genus *Bidens* Linn. in family Asteraceae (with widely disturbed plants. throughout the globe; and 138 genera and 708 species in India) with salient features-Annual or perennial sometimes climbing herbs. Leaves opposite, entire, toothed gashed or 1-2 pinnate. Heads corymbosely panicled or subsolitary, heterogamous and rayed, or homogamous and disciform. Ray-flowers, if present, female or neuter, 1-seriate; lingule spreading, yellow or white. Disk-flowers 2-sexual, fertile, tubular; limb cylindric, 5-fid, Innovlucre campanulate or hemispheric; bracts sub-2-seriate, bases cuneate; outer herbaceous, short or leafy, inner flat membranous. Receptacles flat or convex; pales narrow, nearly flat. Another-cells entire or subsagitate. Style-arms of 2-sexual flowers hairy above; tube short, acute or long and subulate. Achenes 4-gonous or dorsally compressed, linear or cuneiform, often narrowed but not beaked above, Pappus of 2-4 rigid, retrosely hispid bristles or O.

Genus *Bidens* Linn. is represented in various regions by about 50 species, chiefly American (*B. pilosa* Linn. probably of American origin). It has about 230 species of cosmopolitan distribution, abundant in tropical America; annual or perennial herbs and some are weeds, six species in India as 2 confined between 320 meters and 1,980 meters in North Western Himayas, 3-4 species occur throughout India.

Bidens bipinnata Linn. (syn. *B. decompoista* Wall ex Dc, *B. piloss* var. *bipinnata* (Linn.) Hook, f.) is closely allied with *Bidens biternaa* (Lour.) Merr. & Sherif., but it is recognizable by its 2-3. pinnate leaves; whereas *Bidens biternata* is characterized by imparipinnate or rarely 2-pinnate leaves and (perhaps not occurring in country specially in North-West Himalayas).

Three species of *Bidens* Linn. are distinguishable on the basis of various characters, and leaf-characterstics make initial difference. Leaves are 2 3-pinnatipartite in *Bidenss bipinnata* Linn.; whereas the leaves are ternate or imparipinnate to bipinnaste in other two species named as *Bidens biternata* (Lour.) Merr. & Shereff ex Sherff, and *Bidens pilosa* Linn. and these two species further differ in flower and achenes specifically.

Outer involcral bracts linear, acute, ciliate. Heads 10 to 30-flowered. achenes 0.5.2 cm. long, with 2-5 awns of 0.3-0.4 cm. long. Marginal flowers 2-4 or wanting, with 2 to 3-dentate corollas are found in *Bidens biternata.*

Outer involucral bracts spatulate, not ciliate. Heads 20 to 40-flowered. Achenes 0.5-2 mm. 1-8 cm. long, with 2-3 awns of 0.2-0.4 cm. long. Marginal flowers 5-7, with 2 to 5-dentate corollas are found in *Bidens pilosa* Linn.

Leaves 1 pinnate and ligules white in *Bidens biternates* (Lour) Merr. - Sherff. when leaves 2-pinnate and ligules yellow in *Bidens wallichii* DC.

Genus *Bidens* Linn. belongs to Group II Tubuliflorae (juice watery and disc florets tubular) and Tribe V. Heliantheae, and this genus plants have papus of 2-4, persistent, spreading awns and ray florets sterile.

The leaves, flowers achenes, roots and whole plant of Bidens *Bidens* species are medicinally useful.

Bidens biternata (Lour.) Merr. & Sherff is medicnally used in various diseases. Achenes are useful as appetiser in case of loss of appetite and other ailing conditions affecting appetite.

Leaves are useful in cough, cuts, ear comp0laints, eye ailments headache, inflammation, snake bite, sores, wounds and bruises. External application in suitable forms in made may be useful in wounds, sores, eye-ear and cutaneous affections particularly. Flowers are also useful in ear and eye complaints and in treating diarrhoea and similar ailments.

Whole plant is useful in ulcers, skin diseases and leprosy. Roots are used in codition of toothache.

Bidens pilosa Linn., is useful in differnet ailments. Infusion of whole plant is useful for cough. Leaves are considered antipyretic and vulnerary. External application of leaves is made in foul ulcers and swollen glands.

The juice of the leaves is used in eye and ear complaints, and the drops are suitably applied to the organs.

Bidens tripartita Linn. is useful medicinally. Whole plant is used in chronic dysentery and eczema, and similar skin complaints.

Medicinal propetities and action of plant drug - Rasa tikta-kasāya, Vīrya usna, Vipāka kaṭu, Tridoṣasāmaka; and Karma kāsaghna, vraṇaropaṇa, grāhi, stambhana, kaṇḍūghana, kaṇḍūghna, tvacya, jvaraghna, svedajanana, sothahara, dantya, cakṣuṣya, sūlaprasamana, viṣaghna, and dīpana.

Therapeutic indication for external and internal application in Kāsa, jvara, vrana, pāmā, vicarcikā, carmavikāra, granthi-sotha, atisāra, pravāhikā, kṣudhanāsa, agnimāndya, sotha, sirahsūla, dantasula, netraroga, karṇaroga, karṇaroga, duṣṭavraṇa, kṣataja vraṇa and sarpadaṁsa.

Catuṣkāṇḍā, Sanskrit name for plant drug.

3

Cardiospermum halicacabum Linn.

Family : Sapindaceae

Regional names: Kanphuti, Kanphata (Hindi), Nayaphataki, Lataphatkar (Bengla), Karocho (Gujarati), Uhinja, Pallolavam (Himalayam), Valulavse, Mudakkitaam (Tamil), Buddakakara (Telgu); Balloon Vine, winter-cherry (English); Punj-Habul-kalkal, Kanphuta, Kapalphodi, Kolicharmol, Muddakkathan.

Annual-perennial, sarmentose or climbing, glabrous or minutely hairy herbs. Leaves biterrate; uppermost ones often 3-foliolate, leaflets lanceolate-oblong to ovate, decurrent on the periole, acute or obtuse, mucronate at apex, incised-serrate to pinnati-lobed, ciliate, glabrous, except hairy nerves beneath, 1-6 X 0.5-2.5 (-3) cm. Petiole 0.5-5 cm. long, Flowers white, on peduncled, axillary inflorescences with racemiform branches. Peduncle with 2 circinate tendrils at the top. Pedicels 0.2-0.3 cm. long. Sepals suborbicular, glabrate; outer 2 flat, 0.15 X 0.12 cm. long; inner 2 grooved, 0.3 X 0.2 cm. long. Petals obovate-spatulate, retuse, 0.3 cm. long, with pubeacent scales at base. Stamens 3, filaments hairy, 0.15-0.2 cm. long.

Pistillode in male flowers minute. Ovary hairy on the angles. Capsule 3-gonous, subglobose, inflated, short-hairy, 2 X 2.5 cm. Seeds glabrous, smooth.

Flowering and fruiting : July-March

Distribution : Overall the hotter parts of India and in Ceylon, ascending to 4,000 ft. on the Western Himalayas; also in most other tropical and subtropical countries.

Cardiospermum halicacabum Linn.

Annual orr perennial nearly glabrous climbing herb. Stems slender furrowed. Leaves deltoid or ovate, petioled. Leaflets deeply cut, acuminate, glabrous, thin and flaccid. Cymes small, terminating a long stiff slender axillary peduncle, and provided beneath the cyme with 2 opposite circinate tendrils. Flowers very small, white, sepals and petals rounded. Capsule wide, depressed pyriform, trigonous, winged at the angles, valves papery, veined, finely pubescent. Seeds globose, smooth, black; aril heart-shaped, white.

Plant occurring commonly with the area of Upper Gangetic Plains and adjacent regions, climbing on hadges, and over bushes. Flowering, fruiting and fruit-ripening stages during the period ranging from rains to spings in various areas of the region.

Casrdiospermum halicacabum Linn. A Climbing herb. Stem and branches furrowed. Petiole 5-8 cm. long; leaflets ovate, acuminate, up to 5 X 3 cm., glabrescent. Flowers small, yellow. Capsule winged.

Plant distribution in Tropics; southern India, Karnataka. Fairly in Uttar Pradesh and Bengal, and several regions of country. Common in scrub jungles, hedges, forest edges and forest localities in Siwaliks. Herb common during the monsoon period on the Ridge and the neighbouring hilly tracts, often climbing on shrubs and trees in shady places of depressions, Delhi region and adjacent parts, Northern India; and Central India, Madhya Pradesh, Uttar Pradesh and Bihar.

Genus *Cardiospermum* Linn. in family Sapindaceae (about 150 genera with over 2,000 species in tropics and subtropics; and about 19 genera and 45 species in India) with salient features - Climbing herbs with wiry stems and branches. Leaves alternate, biternate, exstipualte; leaflets coarsely dentate. Recemes axillary, lowest pair of pedicels developed into spiral tendrils. Flowers irregular, polygamo-dioecious. Sepals 4, concave, the 2 outer ones smaller. Petals 4, in pairs, the 2 larer lateral ones usually adhering to the sepals, each with an emarginate scale above the base, the 2 smaller inferior and more from the stamens, each furnished with a small crested scale. Disk unilateral, wavy, almost reduced to 2 round or linear glands opposite the lower petals. Stamens 8, excentric; filaments free or coite, the 3 nearest to the glands shorter than the rest. Ovary 3-celled; style short, 3-fid, ovules solitary. Capsule 3-celled, 3-valved, inflated, loculicidal. Seeds globose, usually arillate at the base, exalbuminous.

There are about 12 or 14 species of the genus *Cardiospermum* Linn. in tropics, with the chief centre in America; and 2 species in India, one in Western and Southern India, and one species in hotter parts of India.

Many plants from Siwalik region are referable to *Cardopsermum halicacabum* Linn. var *halicacahum* Linn. which is characterised by smaller fruits in contrast to larger fruits of *C. halicacabum* Linn. var. *luridum* (Bl.) Adelb.

Casriospermum Linn. is primarily separated from several other genera plants in family Sapindaceae as *Cardpospermum* plants have climbing herbaceous habit and leaves biternate particularly, as plants of *Cardiospermum* are specifically climbing herbs and various other genera are of trees, shrubs or any other similar habit in general.

The roots, leaves, seeds and whole plant of *Cardiospermum halicacabum* Linn. are medicinally useful.

Roots and leaves are diuretic, laxative, stomachic, alternative and emetic, externally used as a rubefacient.

Whole plant in rheumatism, stiffness of limits and snake bite. Roots are diaphoretic, diuretic, aperient, laxative, rubifacient, emmenagogue. Roots are also useful in rhemuatism, lumbago and nervous diseases.

Leaves are rubifacient and useful as poultice for rheumatic complaints. Juice of leaves is used as cure agianst earache.

Plant contains saponin and roots are all chemically potent.

The alcoholic extact of fat-free residue left after petroleum other ex-traction of air dried plant, yeilded a crystalline product m.p. 150°, which formed an acetate with pyridine and acetic anhydride. The compound was identified as stigmasterol which was probably present in the form of a glycoside.

The presence of B-sitosterol, phlophene and phlobatannin in the roots of Indian samples is reported. Previous chemical work on the plant *Cardiospermum halicacbum* Linn. report the presence of anebrachitol, which is a monomethyl ether of inositol, B-sitosterol and the presenc eof a saponin or saponins. From the acetone extract of the raw material, quebrachitol was isolated in poor yield. Isolation of a proanthocyanidin and apigenin from the alcoholic extract and their characterisation by chemical and physical methods are reported.

The material examined for its polyphenolic constituents, proanthocyanidins could not be detected but apigenin was isolated and characterised by chemical, spectral and chromato-graphic methods. It occurs in plant in combination with glucose. The presence of saponins indicated by chemical screening could not be substantiated in either batch of the material.

Leaves of the plant are useful in anasarca, earache, eye-sore, lungs diseases, stiffness of limbs, wounds, biliousness and rheumatism. Leaves are also used to wounds.

Stems are useful in fever. Roots are useful in eye complaints, lungs disorders, rheumatism, limbs stiffness, earache, dizziness and other ailments.

Seeds are useful in earache, eye sores, rheumatism and limbs stiffness, and other ailments. Whole plant is useful in nervine complaints, fever and rheumatism.

Roots are edible.

Plant is also useful in veterinary medicine. Roots are used in lice of cattles.

Pharmacological observations find that the essential oil obtained from the seeds of plant show an immediate fall in blood pressure of anaesthesized dogs, lasting for an hour and a half. Atropinization does not alter the effect of the essential oil. Lower doses of the oil (20-100 meg.) causes a marked stimulation of isolated frog's heart. It causes an increase in the tone of isolated rabbit's intestine. Higher doses completely relaxed the intestines.

A prolonged hypotensive effect in anaesthesized dogs is caused with water soluble fraction of the dried alcoholic extract of seeds obtained from this plant. It was not affected by pretreatment with atropine sulphate. It causes an inhibitation of movement of isolated rabbit's intestines. An initial depression followed by marked stimulation in isolated frog's heart preparation is observed with the water soluble portion of the extract.

Medicinal properties and action - Rasa katu-tikta, Vīrya Uṣṇa, vīpāka katu, Guṇa tiksna-snigdha -sara, Vātakaphahara (tridoṣa-sāmaka); and Karma jvaraghna, vranaropaṇa mūtrala, sāraka, dīpana, vāmaka, rasāyana, vedanāsthāpana, nāḍībalya, sothahara, svedajanana, cakṣuṣya, mārdavakara, snehana and visaghna.

Therapeutic indication in vraṇa, netraroga, karṇasūla, jvara, āmavāta, vātavyādhi, sotha, urahvikāra, nāḍīdaurbalya, pittavikāra, sarpaviṣa, mutravikāra, vibandha, netravaikara and other various ailments.

Pasucikitsā - pasukrimi - likṣā

Khādya - mula

Karnasphoṭā, Indravallī and Sphoṭṭalatā, Samkrit names or the plant drug.

4

Ceropegia bulbosa Roxb.

Ceropegia acuminata Roxb.

C. bulbosa var. *esculenta* (Edge) Hook. f.

C. bulbosa var. *lushii* (Graham) Hook. f.

Family : Asclepiadacae

Regional names : Khaparhadu (Hindi), Patal-alumbari (Bombay), Galot (Punjabi), Palatige (Telgu); Kendua, Khantondi.

Twining pernnial herb; rootstock tuberous, somewhat flattened like a turnip emitting many from below. Stems very slender, usually glabrous. Leaves extremely variable, petioled and upto 2 in. long, the lowest almost orbicular, the upper elliptic-ohlong or obovate, usually apiculate and with a rounded truncate, subcordate or acute base. Flowers few, in peduncled, umbellate cymes; peduncle up to i in. long; pedicels much shorter. Calyx-segments R̄ in. long, lanceelate, acute. Corolla less than 1 in. long, greenish, tube inflated at the base; lobes small liner from a traingular base, violet purple and villous within. Outer corolla tube 4, minute, inner filiform. Folicles about 4 in. long, terete, tapering to a slender point glabrous. Seeds 1/3 in. long. ovate-oblong, flat.

Flowering and fruiting : Hot season

Distribution : Punjab Plain and southwards to Travancore.

Ceropegia bulbosa Roxb.

Rhizome tuberous; stem trailing. Leaves ovate, glabrous, 3-6 cm. long; slightly cordaste, fleshy. Cymes 3-5-flowered. Corolla about 2.5 cm. long, whitish-green, purple striate; lobes narrow, short, densely purple pilose. Outer corona lobes rounded to shortly acute, glabrous, equalling the gynostregium; inner lobes straight, clavate.

Plant occurring in the Doab of Upper Gangetic Plains, and in Bundelkhand also Delhi area in, and in adjoining region, Punjab; Northern and Central India.

Ceropegeia bulbosa Roxb. A twining, slender herb. Leaves very variable, upto to 5 x 1.5 cm. Flowers violet-purple, few, in peduncled, umbellate cymes. Corolla tube inflated at the base.

Plant occurring in Southern India; Konkan, South Canara, Malabar, Deccan and Carnatir; occasional along roadsides in middle Shiradi Ghats, Karnataka. Plant flowering in October or autumn season.

Ceropegia tuberosa Roxb.

Ceropegia candelabrum auct. non L.

Family : Ascelepiadaceae

Regional names: Patalatumbi (Hindi), Khap-parkadu (Bombay), Bachaimandu (Telgu); Bhutumbi.

Rhizome tuberous; stem twining. Leaves ovate to lanceolate, sparsely hispid, 3-7 cm. long, base acute to slightly cordate, apex acuminate to mucronate. Cymes mostly 5-15-flowerd. Corolla 2-4 cm. long, whitish-green, purple-striate; mouth slightly dilated; lobes narrow, densely purple-pilose. Outer corona lobes spatulate, about 3 times the length of the outer. Gynostegium stipiate.

Flowring and fruiting : June - October

Distribution : Central and Southern Peninsular India; Sri Lanka

Ceropegia candelabrum L. ssp. *tuberosa* (Roxb.) Huber.

Ceropegia tuberosa Roxb.
Ceropegia candelabrum Linn.
Family : Asclepiadaceae

Rhizome tuberous; stem twining. Leaves usually ellipitc, glabrous, slightly apiculate. Corolla swollen at base; crown narrower, ending in a short, brownish-purple beak. Follicles up to 10 cm., narrowly attenuate.

Flowering and fruiting : October

Plant occurring in Southern India; wet deciduous forests, Karnataka.

Ceropegia elegans Wall.

Ceropegia mysorensis Wight.

C. walkerae Wight.

Family : Asclepiadaceae

Rhizome not tuberous, stem twining. Leaves elliptic, glabrous or slightly puberulent, 3-12 cm. long, base rounded, apex slightly acuminate. Cymes mostly 2-4-flowered. Corolla 2-4 cm. long, dark purple; mouth widely dilated; lobes broad and folded back upon themselves, long purple-ciliate on the margins. Outer corona lobes, deeply bifid; pilose on the margins, extending above the gynostegium inner lobes linear; less than 2 times the length of the outer. Gynostegium sessile.

Flowring and fruiting : September - March.

Distribution : Southern Peninsular India and Sri Lanka

Ceropegia hirsuta Wight. & Arn.

Family : Asclepiadaceae

Rhizome tuberous, stem twining. Leaves variable, mostly ovate-elliptic, with a rounded base, pilose; apex acute. Cymes 1-4-flowered. Corolla 3-4.5 cm. long, greenish-white outside and purple-striate inside; mouth slightly dilated; lobes linear, densely long purple-pilose within at the base, glabrous above. Outer corona lobes deltoid with cleft apex, long plilose, extending above the gynostegium; inner lobes linear and hooked at the tips, 3 times the length of the outer. Gynostegium short-stipiate.

Flowering and fruiting : July - October

Distribution : Southern Gangetic Plain southward to Karnataka. Common in western plan and dry decidous forests.

Ceropegia spiralis Wight.

Family : Asclepiadaceae

Rhizome tuberous; stem erect. Leaves narrowly linear, glabrous, 10-20 cm. long. base and apex acute. Cymes mostly single flowered. Corolla 4-6 cm. long, greenish-purple below and purple above; mouth slightly dilated; lobes linear to ovate, purple-pilose within nearly to the apex. Outer corona lobes entire to slightly bifid, glabrous, inner lobes linear. Gynostegium sessile.

Flowering and fruiting : August - September

Southern Peninsular India; Karnatka.

Distribuion:

Ceropegia elegans Wall.

Ceropegia mysorensis Wight.

C. walkerae Wight.

Family : Asclepiadaceae

Rhizome not tuberous, stem twining. Leaves elliptic, glabrous or slightly puberulent, 3-12 cm. long, base rounded, apex slightly acuminate. Cymes mostly 2-4-flowered. Corolla 2-4 cm. long, dark purple; mouth widely dilated; lobes broad and folded back upon themselves long purple-ciliate on the margins. Outer corona lobes deeply bifid, pilose on the margins, extending above the gynostegium; inner lobes linear, less than 2 times the length of the outer. Gynostegium sessile.

Flowering and fruiting : September - March

Distribution : Southern Peninsular India and Sri Lanka. Karnataka, fairly common in Ghats.

Ceropegia wallichi Wight.

Family : Asclepiadaceae

Pubescent, exrect shrub. Leaves shortly stalked, ovate, obtuse or acute. Flowers dark red purple, axillary or in small clusters. Base of the corolla-tibe dilated, mouth funnel shaped, lobes erect; coronal scales 10 in twp series, often united in a short 10 lobed cup, adnate to the staminal tube. Follicle smooth, long pointed.

Flowering and fruiting : April.

Distribution : Temperate regions from Simla (Shimla), Himachal Pradesh to Nepal; Kumaon, U.P.

Some other relevant species of *Ceropegia* Linn. may be indicated especially from India and adjacent regions.-

Ceropegia fimbrilifera Bedd.

Rhizome tuberous, stem erect. Plant in Southern Peninsular India. Plant flowering in October; Karnataka.

Ceropegia juncea Roxb.

Rhizome not thickened, stem twining. Plant in Peninsular India. Plant flowering in December - August; Karnataka.

Ceropegia candelabrum L. var. **biflora** (L.) Ansari

Ceropegia tuberosa Roxb.

Ceroplegia media (Huber) Ansai

Ceropegia evasti var. media Huber.

Ceropegia vincaefolia Hook.

Ceropegia hirsuta var. *vincaefolia* (Hook). f.

C. stocksi Hook. f.

C. polyantha Blatt. & McCann.

Ceropegia angustifolia Wt. A slender, perennial twining herb, with fasciculated, fusiform tuberous roots. Plant in Siwaliks, scrub-jungles, ravine-slopes and forest-edges. Plant flowering during July to October period.

Ceropegia macrantha Wight. An extensive rather stout nearly glabrous climber. Tropical Himalayas from Kumaon to Sikkim. Plant flowering and fruiting from July to November.

Genus *Ceropegia* Linneaus in family Asclepiadaceae (about 130 genera and 2,000 species widely spread throughout the tropical; the tropical and subtropical regions of the world) with salient features - Twining, rarely erect, perennial herbs, often with a tuberous rootstock. Leaves opposite, sometimes minute or none. Flowers in lateral peduncled usually umbellate cymes, rarely solitary, often large, white or greenish-and purple. Calyx 5-partite, lobes narrow. Corolla-tube elongate, straight or curved, often swollen at the base; lobes erect or incurved and with cohering tips, often at length recurved or reflexed, valvate in bud. Corona staminal, double, attached to the column;

outer cupular, entire or toothed; inner more or less adnate to outer, consisting of 5 lobes erect or incumbent over the anthers. Staminal columns very short, adnate to the base of corolla; anthers stout without appendages; pollen-masses one in each cell, short, erect or ascending, attached to the pollen - carriers by short caulicles or subessile. Stigma included, truncate or shortly conical. Follicles usually slender, acuminate, smooth, Seeds coinose.

There are 50 or more species in the genus *Ceropegia* Linn., in tropical and Temperate Asia and Africa, also in Malaya and Mauritius; or about 150 species in Canary Islands, tropical and South Africa, Madagascar, tropical and subtropical Asia and North queensland; and about 43 species in India, chiefly in the mountains of Southern and Western India, with a few in the Himalaya.

In the family Asclepiadacae, the genus *Ceropegia* Linn. is of twining stems and tubular corolla in twining plants, procumbent or straggling, generally, with leaves absent or reduced and caducous, leaves well developed, lanceolate in linear, rootstock tuberous and corollas tubular. Plants are twiners or climbers - leafy twiners - of *Ceropegia* plants with flowers violet-purple.

Generally they are twiner, straggling or climbing plants, sometimes erect herbs, with watery sap. Cymes ubmbellate, lateral. Corolla tubular, lobes valvate, Corona of 2 series of lobes, the outer sometimes deeply bifid, the inner entire. Gynostegium stipitate or sessile. Pollinia erect from dark horny corpuscula 2 per anther, waxy, with pellucid margins.

Two new species of genus *Ceropegia Linn.* are distinguishable on the basis of flower characters. For the instance, the corolla-lobes ciliate with 0.7-1 cm. long, purple in *Ceropegia borii* Raizada; whereas corolla-lobes eciliate in *Ceropegia raizadiana* Babu.

Various species of genus *Ceropegia* Linn. differ of characters and habit. Leaves are poorly developed or absent and stems fleshy in *Ceropegia juncea* Roxb., when several other species of *Ceropegia* Linn. have well developed leaves and stems are not fleshy.

Mostly species are of twining stems with linear leaves, if present, on upper stem only. Various species are separated for different characterstics. For the instance, the plants are densely pilose, especially on the stems and peduncles and inner corona lobes hooked in *Cerpegia hirsuta* Wight. & Arn.; whereas the plants are sparsely pubescent or glabrous and inner corona lobes not hooked in some other species, carrying difference in other characters. Leaves fleshy in *Coropegia bulbosa* Roxb. when leaves are membranous or subcoriaceous in a few other species. Corolla funnel-shaped in *Ceropegia elegans* Wall. when corolla not funnel-shaped in other species. Crown of corolla lobes forming short and blunt beak in *Ceropegia candelabrum* L.; whereas crown of corolla lobes drawn out in *Ceropegia tuberosa* Roxb.

Sometimes *Ceropegia tuberosa* Roxb. are *Ceropegia candelabrum* L. are similar (reduced or synonymous); but these two species are quite distinct especially with regard to the corolla lobes, and the crown of the corolla lobes is shortly beaked in the latter and elongate-spatulate in the former.

Ceropegia raizadiana Babu is morphologically interesting and closely allied to *Ceropegia. angustifolia* Wt. or *Ceropegia macrantha* Wt. (rather earlier as anyone species), but it is recognizable from the former by much broader, ovate leaves, curved corolla-tube with a swollen base, lanceolate corolla-segments and 5-deeply 2-fid coronal scales; and from the latter by corolla-segments being connate at the top, deely 2-fid coronal scales, linear sepals and petiole with basal and apical glands.

Coropegia borii Raizada is related to *C. hirsuta* w. & A. var. *stenophylla* Hk. f., but it can be distinguished from it chiefly by the practically glabrous leaves and the characterstic hemispherical head fringed with long purple hairs.

The tubers of *Ceropegia species* are mainly medicinally useful.

The tubers of *Ceropegia bulbosa* Roxb. are tonic and digestive. Alkaloid caropegine is the bitter principle of the tuberous root.

The tubers of *Ceropegia tuberosa* Roxb. are tonic in the bowel complaints of children, cure for dysentery and and diarrhoea. Tubers are edible.

The tubers of *Ceropegia hirsuta* Wt. & Arn. are edible.

The tubers of *Ceropegia bulbosa* Roxb, are refrigerant, edible and useful for vitality. Tubers and leaves are edible and also used as vegetable.

The tubers of *Ceropegia candelabrum* L. are useful in bowel complaints of children.

The tubers of *Ceropegia candelabrum* L. var. *biflora* (L.) Ansari (*C. tuberosa* Roxb.) are edible and useful as vegetable.

The tubers of *Caropegia lawii* Hook f. are edible and useful as vegetable.

The tubers of *Ceroplegia oculata* Hook. f. are edible.

The tubers of *Ceropegia panchganensis* Blat. & Mc Cann. are edible.

Mostly all the parts of plant *Ceropegia bulbess* Roxb. are edible in certain areas, either raw or stewed in their curries or other similar preparations of vegetable or alike for eating purpose. Fresh roots are tasting like a raw turnip, and the leaves and stem like pursalane.

The tuberous roots or fleshy underground parts of most of these species are stated to be eaten by animals in forests, apparently by wild boars and others.

Medicinal properties and action of plant drug -

Kandalatā, the Sanskrit name for the plant drug.

5

Cleistanthus collinus Benth.

Lebidioropsis orbicularris Muell. - Arg.

Cluytia collinus Roxb.

Cleistanthus collinus (Roxb) Benth. Hook. f.

Family : Euphorbiaceae

Regional names: Garari (Hindi), Karljuri (Bengal), Nilappulai (Tamil), Kandishe (Telgu), Odaichi (Tamil); Garari, Karada, Parashi.

Small trea with a dark rough bark; branches stiff, smooth or postulate. Leaves coriaceous, 1-1/4 -4 in. long, orbicular, broadly obovate or elliptic, rounded or retuse at the apex, glabous beneath; pale when dry; main lateral nerves 6-8 pairs; very slender; petiole 1/4 in., slender. Flowers in small axillary and shortly spicate villous clusters. Calyx 1/4 in. diam., ovate-lanceolate. Petals narrow, fleshy, incurved. Disk of male flowers pulvinate; of the females conical with a thick margin. Ovary globose, glabrous; styles free, thick; stigmas lobed. Capsule sessile, wrinkled, rounded, small, obscurely 3-lobed, dark-brown, shining and wrinkled when dry. Seeds 1/8 in. in diam, globose, reddish-brown.

Flowering and fruiting : Summers to winters

Distribution : Central Provinces mm. Chota Nagpur and Circars to Southern India, and Ceylon.

Genus *Cleistanthus* Hook. f. in family Euphorbicaeae (about 4,000 species throughout the world, chiefly tropical and excepting in Arctic regions) with salient features - Trees or shrubs. Leaves alternate, bifarious, entire. Flowers monoecious, small or minute, in axillary clusters or spikes, all sessile or the females shortly pedicelled. Male flowers : Calyx-segments 5, valvate. Petals 5, short, scale-like, stalked or spathulate. Disk broad, entire or sinuate. Stamens 5; filaments connate below in a central column, bearing a pyramidal or 3 - lobed pistilode, free and spreading above; anther-cells parallel. Female flowers : Disk double, the inner conic or turbinate, more or less enclosing the young ovary. Ovary 3 (rarely 4) - celled, usually clothed with long hairs; ovules 2 in each cell; styles 3, free, 2-fid. Fruit a sessile or stipitate subglobose or depressed capsule with three 2- or scanty; cotyledons thin or flesh often folded.

Genus *Cleistanthas* Hook. f. is with species about 30, in Tropical India, Malaya and Africa.

Genus *Cleistanthus* Hook.f. is among the genera having flowers dioecious or monoecious; infloroescence mostly axillary or lateral; perianth of sepals always present and sometimes also petals. Leasves simple, usually entire. Two genera bear male flowers in axillary fascicles or soliary in the axils, namely *Bridela* Wild. and *Clesitanthus* Hook. f. and they commonly have corolla of 5 (rarely 6) scale-like petals; and *Clesitanthus* Hook. f. is separable for its 3-celled ovary, fruits a capsule and small deciduous trees, in comparison to *Bridelia* Willd. having 2-celled ovary, indehiscent fruit and trees or scandent shrubs. Corolla is absent in both sexes and sepals imbricate in many other genera of family, keeping genus *Clesistanthus* distinct.

Some other species of the genus *Cleistanthus* Hook. f. may be indicated :

Cleeistanthus refus (Hook. f.) Gehrm.

Bridelia rufa Hook. f.

Cleistanthus sumatranus (Miq.) Muell.-Arg.

Leiopyxis sumatrana Miq.

Celeistanthus heterophylus Hook. f.

C. laevis Hook. f.

Cleistanthus collinus (Roxb.) Benth & Hook. f. syn. *Cluytia colling* Roxb. is occurring in forests of Bundelkhand in Uttar Pradesh Madhya Pradesh, Bihar, Orissa, North Circars, Karnataka, and the Deccan especially Hyderabad and Malabar.

The bark, roots, leaves and fruits of *Cleistanthus collinus Benth.* are medicinally useful. The plant is extremely poisonous. The capsules as well as the leaves and roots are very poisonous.

Plant is astringent and extremely poisonous. Extract of leaves roots and especially fruits are violent are considered useful in violent gasto-intestinal irritation and disorders.

Roots, leaves and bark are fish poison.

Stem bark is abortifacient. Roots are considered useful to boils. Stem bark and leaves are useful in skin diseases. Stem bark in useful in wounds.

In veterinary medicine, the leaves are useful in sore of feet in cattles. Leaves are fatal to domestic animals and harmful. Green leaves are insect repellant; and stem is insects resistant.

The bark yields d and fruits give tan. Plant is also employed in charm to drive away the evil in human beings. Plant is used for arrow poison.

The chemical examination of the petroleum ether extract of the fruits shows the pessence of sterol and titerpenoids, apart from tannins, in the alcohol extract. The non-saponifiable fraction when chromatograohed over neutral alumina give two compounds with m.p. 183-87° and 123-

127°. These appear to be luperol and B-sitosterol acetate respectively.

The acetone extract of the leaves furnished ellagic acid, m.p. 360°, and a new lactone named collinusin m.. 196°, molecular formula $C_{21}H_{18}O_8$. Its UV spectrum was similar to that of Y-apopicropodphyllin. Zeisel determination shows the presence of two methoxyl groups and a positive chromotropic acid test supported the presence of a methylene dioxy group. The structure of collinusin is also provided.

Dehydrogenation of collinusin with palladised charcol yields optically inactive dehydrocollinusin, m.p. 235-236°. Its NMR spectrum shows the presence of two methoxyl groups, a methylene-dioxy group and six aromatic protons. Its structure has been determined. The physical properties of dehydrocollinusin resemble those of justicidin B.

Diphyllin is isolated alongwith other compounds from the leaves. It was first isolated from *Diphylleia grayi* roots and the hence the name is given. The structure for diphyllin as well as justicidin has been revised. Diphyllin, m.p. 291°, on drastic oxidation with aqeous alkaline permanganate gives albeit in low yield and 3, 4-methylenedioxybenoic acid,.

Ellagic acid, diphyllin and two new lignan lactones, collinusin and cleistanthin have been isolated from *Clestitanthus collinus.* The major constituent of the leaves is a highly toxic glycoside cleistanthin, mm. 135-136°. Its NRM spectrum shows the presence of five aromatic protons, a mothylenedioxy group, a methylene and four methoxyls.

Cleistanthin, a glycoside isolated from the acetone extract of the leaves, produced consistent increase of neutrophilic granulocyte (NGC) on administration by various routes in rats, mice, cats and monkeys. The rise in NGC is noticed after single oral dose which persists up to 72-120 hours. in different species. i.p. and i.v. injections of glycoside result in the remarkable increase of NGC by 6 hours after injection which reaches to normal values in 24 hours.

Repeated administration of 0.25 mg./kg. per day orally to rats for 30 days mainained the neutrophilic count of a high level without any toxic side effect. Granulocytopenia induced by I.P. injection of cyclophosphamide could be prevented by the glycoside, and the therapeutic index was found to be 12 mg/kg. in the rats under experiments.

Leucopenia was induced in rats (70 mg./kg.) and mice (200 mg./kg.) by a single I.P. injection of cyclophosphamide and after oral dose of 2.5 mg/kg. of cleistanthin, the NGC was significnatly higher, six of seven times more than that of control rats under test.

The alcoholic extract of the whole plant *Gleintanthus collinus* showed anti-cancer activity against human epidermal carcinoma of the nasopharynx in tissue culture.

The medicinal properties and action of the plant drug - Rasa takta-kaṣāya, vīrya uṣṇa, Vipāka kaṭu, Guṇa laghu-tikṣṇa-uṣṇa; Vātakaphahara; Karma vraṇaropaṇa, grāhi, tīkṣṇviṣa and māraka.

Therapeutic indication in vraṇa,kṛmi-kīṭa (rakṣaka) carmavikāra and Karkaṭārbuda (cancer), and other ailing conditions, but with precaution due to severe poisonousness (tīvra viṣāktta).

Bhutavida pṛayoga - phala

Viṣavigyāna - phala, patra, mūla admpaapa.

Saraviṣa pādapa

Pasucikitsā - Pāda vrana, māraka-ghāTaka; matsyaniṣūdana

Mahāgara, Kīṭāri and Bhūttāri, the Sanskrit names for the plant drug.

6

Dipteracanthus prostratus (Poir.) Nees.

Ruellia prostrata Poi.

Dipteracanthus dejectus Nees.

Ruellia wightiana wall.

Ruellia repens Heyne.

Ruellia prostrata Poit. (incl. var. *dejecta* (Nees) Clarke.

Family : Acanthaceae

Regional names : Kalighawani (Gujarati), Upudali (Malayalam), Pottahanchi (Tamil)

Protrate to decumbent-ascending, multicauline, perennial herbs, with a woody base. stems simple or sparingly branched, patently hairy inwards the apex. Leaves ovate-lanceolate, rounded or subconate at base, subacute or subobtuse at apex, subentire-repand, ciliate, glabrate or thinly appressed-setose, lineolate with raphides, 2-8 x 1.5-4 cm. Petiole 2-3 cm. long. Flowers subsessile, solitary Bracteoless obovate - spatulate, subacute, appressed, pubescent, 1-2 cm. long. Calyx 1 cm. long, segments lanceolate, ciliate. Corolla pale-purple, hairy on the outside, 2.5-3 cm. long; lobes rounded-suborbicular. Styles linear, 1.5 cm. long, Capsule densely pubescent, 1.8-2 cm, long.

Flowering and fruiting : March - June, December - April, June-September, or several months of the year.

Distribution : Throughout India from the Punjab and Assam to Ceylon extending to East Africa, Central and Peninsular India.

Ruellia prostrata Lamk. var, *dejecta* Clarke. Small diffuse under shrub. Stems 6-18 in long, prostrate or climbing, amongst bushes, much branched, internodes long, the nodes more or less hairy and often tinged with purple. Leaves up to 3 in. long, ovate or elliptic, acute at both ends, entire, glabrous or slightly hairy, with petioles. Flowers subsessile, solitary or few together; bracteoles similar to the leaves but rhizome. Leaves petioled, lanceolatte ciliate or oblanceolate, the lower one usually smaller and often suborbicular, obtuse or subacute, entire, villous with white hairs on both surfaces especially on the nerves and veins beneath, margins ciliate. Flowers solitary, terminal subsessile; bracteoles resembling the leaves but smaller and narrower, 3/4 in. long, stalked. Calyx-segments 1/4 in. long, linear, puberulous or nearly glabrous. Corolla white up to 2 in. long, tube slender, limb subregular. Capsule 1.5 in. long, oblong, glabrous, often tinged with purple. Seeds few.

Flowering and fruiting :	April to July; Rainy season. Flowers open at sunset and drop off on the following morning.
Distribution :	North and West Bengal and in Chota Nagpur, Upper Gangetic Plains also in Upper Burma.

Ruellia suffruticosa Roxb. An erect pubescent, straggling undershurb. Internodes long. Leaves ellliptic, obovate or oblanceolate, villous with white hairs on both surfaces especially on the nerves and veins beneath; *Dipteracanthus prostratus* (Poir.) Nees. Procumbent herbs. petiole hairy; blade 2.5-4.4 X 1-2.1 cm., ovate, acute, sparsely hairy. Flower axillary, solitary, subsessile; bracts foliaceous, up to 1 X 0.5 cm., ovate. Calyx lobes lanceolate, acute, hairy. Corolla lilac, externally hairy, up to 1.5 cm., segmented into 5 semi-orbicular lobes. Staminodes 0. Seeds flat, discoid.

Plant occurring in Southern India; Karnataka and other various regions; Deccan Peninsula, extending North to Bihar.

Dipteracanthus suffruticosus (Roxb.) Voigt.

Ruellia suffruticosus Roxb.

Ruellia repens - Wall.

Dipteracanthus sibus Nees.

Ruellia suffruticosa Roxb.

Family : Acanthaceae

Regional names : Chaulia, Ranuran (Santals.); Carpondu, Sirrkabel.

Erect pubescent undershrub, 1-2 ft. high. Roots stout, often with fusiform swellings. Stems herbaceous, annually produced from a short creeping woody rhizome. Leaves petioled, lanceolatte ciliate or oblanceolate, the lower one usually smaller and often suborbicular, obtuse or subacute, entire, villous with white hairs on both surfaces especially on the nerves and veins beneath, margins ciliate. Flowers solitary, terminlal subsessile; bracteoles resembling the leaves but smaller and narrower, 3/4 in. long, stalked. Calyx-segments 1/4 in. long, linear, puberulous or nearly glabrous. Corolla white, up to 2 in. long, tube slender, limb subregular. Capsule 1.5 in. long, oblong, glabrous, often tinged with purple. Seeds few.

Flowering and fruiting : April to July; Rainy season. Flowers open at sunset and drop off on the following morning.

Distribution : North and West Bengal and in Chota Nagpur, Upper Gangetic Plains also in Upper Burma.

Ruellia suffruticosa Roxb. An erect pubescent, straggling undershurb. Inter nodes long. Leaves eiliptic, obovate or oblanceolate, villous with white hairs on both surfaces especially on the nerves and veins beneath; margins ciliate. Flowers white, solitary, axillary or more. Corolla and style caducous. Capsules glabrous.

Plant occurring in the areas of Upper Gangetic Plains, Rohilkhand, Siwalikas, North Oudh, Uttar Pradesh, Central and Northern-India, Madhya Bharat, Bihar, Orissa and other areas including Delhi and adjoining parts.

Dipteracanthus patulus (Jacq.) Nees

Ruellia patula Jacq.

Dipteracanthus erectus Nees.

Petalidium patulum Dalz. & ibs.

Family : Acanthaceae

Regional name :

Small hoary-pubescent shrub. Stems erect of long and straggling much-branched, densely and closely pubescent. Leaves .5-1.5 in. long, ovate or elliptic, obtuse and sometimes apiculate, rounded at the base or abruptly narrowed closely pubescent on both sufaces, petioles 1/4-3/4 in. long. Flowers subsessile, solitary or 2-3 together in the axils; bracteoles leaflike, less than 1/2 in. long (incl. the short flat stalk). elliptic, obtuse, densely pubescent and ciliate. Calyx 5-partite, 1/4 in. long, densely pubescent, segments linear-lanceolate, very acute. Corolla pale greyish-pupple, 1-1/4 in. long; hairy outside; tube narrowly cylindric below funnel-shaped above;l lobes 1/4 in. long elliptic or suborbicular. Ovary glabrous except the lip, style hairy. Capsule 1/2-3/4 in. long, clavate, glabrous. Seeds suborbicular nearly glabrous, but with a dense fringe of hair on the margin.

Flowering and fruiting :	Hot and rainy season
Distribution:	Punjab Plain, Rajputana, Sind and southwards through the drier

portions of Western and Southern India to Ceylon, extedning to Arabin, Tropical africa, Abyssinia and Ava.,

Dipteracanthus patulus (Jacq.) Nees. A hoary pubescent, erect or straggling, much-branched undershrubs. Leaves ovate to elliptic, obtuse, hairy. Flowers pale purple, solitary or 2-3 together, cylindric-funnelform. Capsules clavate, glabrous.

Plant occurring in Upper Gangetic Plains; common in uncultivated ground, chiefly in the drier western plortion of the area, Bundelkhand, Merwar and in the ravine tracts skirting the Brijbhumi region in Uttar Pradesh; Delhi area and adjoining parts in the region; common on the Ridge in depressions and also in other parts.

Ruellia patula Jacq. Hoary pubescent herb. Leaves ovate, bracteoles spathulate elliptic or petioled ovate foliaceous.

Dipteracanthus beddomei (Clarke) Sarap.

Ruellia beddomei Clarke:- *Ruellia cornus* Anders (partly, not of Roxb.

Family : Acanthaceae

Erect, multicauline simple or sparingly branched, perennial herb with a woody base. Roots fleshy, fasciculated. Stems 4-gonous, glabrous downwards, apressed, hairy towards the apex. Leaves ovate-elliptic or lanceolate-oblong with a slightly oblique, acute or rounded base, often decurrent, sharply acute or acuminate, sub-entire-undulate, ciliate, appressed-setose, 10-15 X 3.5-5 cm. with 6-7 (-8) pairs of lateral nerves; petiole, 2-3 cm. long. Flowers on 0.3-0.5 cm. long pedicels, bracteoles on 0.6-0.8 cm. long stalks, leaf-like, ovate, subacute 3.5-4 X 1.3-1.5 cm., calyx 0.7-0.8 (-1) cm. long, segments linear-lanceolate, ciliate, corolla, pale-purple, hairy outside, about 8 cm. long, lobes oblong, obtuse 1.8-2 cm., long; style ciliate; Capsule 2.2-2.5 cm. long; reticula 0.3-0.4 cm. long.

Flowers and frutining :	October - December
Distribution :	Central India, Madhya Pradesh, Uttar Pradesh, Orissa.

Plant is shaded and dry localities of forest clearnings, Siwalkis and other regions.

Ruellia beddomei Clarke. Perennial; leaves elliptic acute hairy on both surfaces, bracteoles subpetioled ovate acute leaf-like, sepals 1/2 in., corolla 3 in.

Genus *Dipteracanthus* Nees *emend.* Bremek. sometimes considered congeneric with *Ruellia* Linn. After revision of the genus *Ruellia* Linn., most of the genera assign to genus *Dipteracanthus* Nees. The genus *Ruellia sensu stricto* is represented (in India) by an introduced plant *Ruellia tuberosa* Linn. Another plant is *Ruellia neolongifolius* B. & R. syns. *R. longifolia* (Stocks) T. & J., *Dipteracanthus longifolius* Stocks.

Genus *Dipteracantthus* Nees. (ten species in tropical East Africa, Asia and Australia; and seven species in India, mostly in Southern, Central and Eastern India) with salient features—Herbs. Inflorescences axillary, of 1-2 flowers; bracts folicaeous, exceedng calyx; bracteoles small. Calyx lobes 5. Corolla 5-lobed. Stamens 4, didynamous, not exerted; anthers cells 2, parallel, not spurred; staminodes occasionally present. Locules 3-6-ovuled. Capsule clavate. Seeds compressed, usually hairy.

Genus *Dipteracanthus* in family Acanthaceae (species upwards of 2,000 in tropical and warm temperate regions) belongs to Tribe 3 Ruelliene and subtribe 1 Polyspreme with general characters - Ovules 3-12 in each cell, capsule normally 6-or more-seeded; and with specific character of sub-equally 5-lobed corolla in *Ruellia* Linn. and other some co-genera in Polyspermore.

Dipteracanthus prostratus (Poir) Nees, *D. patulus* (jacq.) Nees and *D. suffruticosus* (Roxb.) Voigt. initially differ on the basis of habit of plants as *D. prostratus* is of prostrate or climbing habit when other two foregoing species are of erect or diffuse habit; and further these may be distinguishable for other characterstics such as *D. prostratus* has ovary and capsule pubescent, and the ovary and capsule glabrous in rest of these two species, but they differ in flower colour as flowers are pale purple in *D. patulus* and flowers white in *D. suffruticosus* besides other characters.

There is characterstic difference between *Dipteracanthus prostratus* (Poir) Nees and *D. beddomei* (Clarke) Santap., such as ovary and capsule are pubescent and corolla 3 long cm. in former species, while latter has glabrous ovary and capsule and corolla 7-7.5 cm. long.

Dipteracanthus beddomei (Clarke) Santap. is closely allied to *D.suffruticosus* (Roxb.) Voigt. but this is easily recognizable by sharply acute leaf-apex, longer calyx and corolla. Another species *D. prostratus* (Poir) Nees plants are variable in habit, size and shape of leaves and size of flowers.

The roots, leaves and while plant of *Dipteracanthus* syn. *Ruellia* species are medicinally useful.

Roots of *Dipteracasnthus suffruticosus* Voigt. are useful in gonorrhoea, syphilis and renal affections. Dried and ground roots are given in a doze of 2 oz. that causes abrotion. This is also used as a remedy for sore eyes.

Roots are considered useful in giving in the stage of abdominal pain after labour in female cases. Plant is considered useful in bronchitis, cough, diarrhoea, fever and dropsy.

Roots are also edible as these are used in local drinks.

The leaves are used with liquid copal as a medicine for gonorrohoea. It is also considered useful in eye diseases.

Medicinal properties and action of plant drug - Rasa tikta-kaṣāya, Vīrya uṣṇa, Vipāka kaṭu, Vātakapha nāsaka (tridoṣa-sāmaka); and Karma kāsahara, tvacya, raktasodhaka, vraṇaropaṇa, mūtrala, sangrāhi, stambhana, garbhyasrāvakara, uttejaka, dīpana, cakṣusya, vedanā-sthāpana and jvaraghna.

Therapeutic indication in jvara, kāsa, svāsa, carmavikāsa, raktavikāra-raktaduṣṭi, vraṇa, phiraṅga, upadaṁsa, netraroga, avasāda, atisāra, pravāhika, agimāndya, ratijaroga and other various diseases.

Romasā, the Sanskrit name for the plant drug.

7

Glossogyne bidens (Retz.) Alston.

Glossogyne pinnatifida DC.

Zinnia bidens Retz.

Family : Asteraceae (Composiate)

Regional names : Kamraj, Baragom, Nakdana; Barangom - bir - barangom (Santhal), pardosibhangra (Gujarati).

Erect, perennial herbs, with a stout, thick, fusiform root. Stems often many from a somewhat woody base, simple or widely branched in the upper part, erect or ascending from the decmbent base, glabrous. Leaves mostly in a radical rosette, petioled, 1 to 2-pinnatipartite or -pinnate; cauline ones very much reduced or smaller; 3-5 (-6) cm. long; segments linear-lanceolate, entire, acute, mucronate, glabrous. Heads solitary, terminal, on 2-5 cm. long peduncles. Involucral bracts 1-seriate, lanceolate, obtuse, glabrous, 0.3-0.4 cm. long. Marginal flowers with yellow. 3-dentate ligules. Corolla of disk-flowers yellow. Achenes black, 0.7-0.8 cm. long. Pappus-bristles 2, retrosely hairy.

Flowering and fruiting : March - November

Distribution : Punjab Plains, West Bengal and south to Madras; Chota Nagpur, North Circars, and Deccan of Madras (Tamilnadu) State.

Glossogyne pinnatifids DC

Erect, fusiform woody. Stems usually may from the root, erect or ascending, 6-18 in. high; branches slender, forked. Leaves usually radical, 1-2 in. (with petiole), pinnatified, triangular; segments few, rigid, linear, acute, glabrous veins prominent beneath. Flowering branches 6-12 in. long with a small, pinnatifid leaf of each fork, stiff, grooved. Heads few, long-peduncled, Invol-bracts linear, obtuse, glabrous. Achenes deeply grooved, black.

Plant fairly common in sandy ground and grassy lands; Upper Gangetic plains, especially along the base of the Himalayas from Dehradun to North Oudh, also in Bundelkhand. Herb flowering during autumn.

Genus *Glossogyne* Creb. in the family Asteraceae (Compositae-coextensive with dicotyledonous vegetation with genera about 1,000 and species over, 8,000) with salient features - Perennial glabrous herbs, with almost naked stems and branches. Leaves radical, crowded, pinnatifid, or cuneate and 3-toothed; cauline alterante, or the lower opposite or 0.

Heads small few, corymbose, heterogamous and rayed, or homogamous and disaform. Ray-flowers female fertile ligules spreading, yellow (or probably white). Disk-flowers 2-sexual, fertile, tubular, limb, 5-fid. Involucre small; bracts 2-3 seriate, narrow, bases connate. Receptacle flat; pales carious. Flat or concave. Anthers-bases obtuse. Style-arms of 2-sexual flowers with long hairy tips. Achenes dorsally compressed, linear, ovoid or almost winged, glabrous, truncate. Pappus of retrosely scabrid bristles.

Genus *Glossogyne* Cass. belongs to the series I Tubuliforae and tribe V Helanthoideae with common features - Heads heterogamous, usually rayed or homogamous and rayless. Ray-flowers female fertile or neuter. Disk-flowers 2-sexual fertile or sterile. Receptacle paleaceous. Anther-bases not tailed. Style-arms of disk-flowers, truncate or appendiculate, of the sterile flowers, not divided. Achenes usually angled. Pappus of 2-5 bristles or paleaceous or O.

Among the genera in general with features. Heads heterogemous and rayed, or homogamous and rayless; ray-flowers fem. or neuter; disk-flowers 2-sexual and fertile, or the inner rarely sterile; receptacles paleaceous; achenes more or less dorsally compressed; pappus or 2-4 awns or 0, has genra *Glossogyne* Cass is distinguished of leaves mostly radical demand achenes with 2 persistent bristles which are spacific characterstics, separating another genus *Chrysathellum* Rich. of leaves usually cauline, alternate and achenes and awned; as the two genera have common characters of style-arms with a long appendage, ray-flowers fertile and leaves pinnatifid or toothed, and both genera *Glossogyne* Cass and *Chrysanthellum* Rich differ by leaf, flower and other characters. In other two genera of this group, the style-arms with a short appendage, for the instance, are in *Glossocardia* Cass and *Bidens* Linn. having other distinguishing characters of leaves, flowers, achenes and others.

The roots, herb and whole plant of *Glossogyne pinnatifida* DC. are medicially useful.

A preparation from the roots of plant is employed in snake-bite and scorpion-sting.

The roots are useful in abdominal pain, boils and bone fractures.

Whole plant is useful as anthelmintic, and in headache and in toothache.

Plant is considered useful against doges bites and rabid dogs. It is also similarly used in jackal bites.

Whole plant is useful in cholera, dysentery, diarrhoea and gastrointestinal disorders.

Whole plant is useful in impotency, spermatorrhoea and similar sexual and seminal complaints.

Plant is useful as a galactagogue, and given for lactation in females.

Whole plant is useful in cough, catarrhal affections and throat ailments.

Whole plant is useful in worms affections.

Plant is useful in spleenic complaints.

Herb is useful in syphilis.

In veterinary medicine, the plant is useful. Whole plant is applied in bone fractures of cattles and other animals. Herb is useful in wounds of birds and similar ailments.

Medicinal properties and action of the plant drug - Rasa tikta-kaṭu-kaṣāya, Vīrya uṣṇa, Vipāka kaṭu; Vāttakaphasāmaka-pittasaṁamana (tridoṣa sāmaka); and Karna viṣaghna, krimighna, varaṇaropana, saṅgrāhi, vedanāsthāpana, Dīpana, pācana, anulomana, āmapācana, sandhānīya, balya, stanyajanane, kācahara, kaphaghna, kaṇṭhya, sukraianana, vṛṣya, dantya, sūlaprasamana, stambḥana, maktaprasādana and kaṇḍūghna.

Therapeutic indication for internal and external uses in Viṣa, jāṅgamaviṣa, vṛṣcikadaṁsa, sarpadaṁsa, srgāldaṁsa, kukkuradaṁsa, udarakrimi, viṣūcikā, vrana, piḍikā, kṣata, carvavikāra, raktadoṣa; plīhavikāra, udarasūla, ratilaroga-phiraṅga, sukrameha, sukradaurbala, napunsakatā, dantasūla, kāsa, kaṇṭharoga, atisāra, āmātisāra, pravāhikā, stanyakṣaya and other ailments.

Pasucikitsā - Asthibhagna and vraṇa (pakṣī)

Kāmarāja, the Sanskrit name for the plant drug.

Glycosmis mauritiana (Lam.) Tanaka

Limonia mauritiana Lank.

L. pentaphylla snesus Hook . Roxb.

L. pentaphylla auct. non Retz.

L. pentaphylla DC.

L. pentaphylla (Retz.) Correa (incorrect)

Glycosmis triphylla Wight.

Family : Rutaceae

Regional names : Bannimbu, Deonba, Golugu

Medium-sized trees. Leaves 5-more foliolate; leaflets ovate-lanceolate, acuminate, rounded at base, up to 12 X 4-6 cm., coricaeous. Inflorescence brown-pubescent. Flowers white (slightly smaller than the other species *Glycosmis arborea)*. Ovary eglandular, sparsely pilose, 5-locular.

Berry ovoid, to 1 cm. across, yellow.

Flowering and fruiting : January - May

Distribution : Southern India and Sri Lanka. Fairly common in Upper Ghats, Karnataka.

Glycosmis arborea (Roxb.) DC

Limonia pontaphylla Retz.

(non *Glycosmis pentayphlla* (roxb.). DC.

Limonia arborea Roxb.

Glycosmis pentaphylla auct. non (Roxb.) DC

G. cochinchinensis auct. excl.

Tolnifera cochinchinensis Lour.

Glycosmis chylocarpa W. & A.

Family : Rutaceae

Regional names:	Ban-nimbu (Hindi), Ashshoura (Bengla), Konji (Tamil),Gonji (Telgu), Kimira (Marathi); Chaulgua, Panal, Karhangwae, Tarang, Taw-shauk (Lower Burma), obok (Upper-Burma).

Small evergreen glabrous shrub. Leaves very variable. usually 3-5-foliolate, rarely 1-foliolate. Leaflets 4-9 in. long, ovate-lanceolate ovate or obovate, obtuse acute or acuminate, penninerved, entire or obscurely crenulate. Flowers small, white-fragrant, in erect terminal or lateral pubescent panicles. Ovary glabrous, covered with projecting glands, usually 5-celled; style very short and stout. Berry small, subglobose or somewhat compressed, white, pink or blue.

Flowring and fruiting :	Greater part or the year.
Distribution :	Tropical and sutropical Himalayas from the Sutlej to Sikkim, ascending to 7,000 fit., Assam, Malaya Peninoula, Southern India and Ceylon; exteeding to China, the Burma, Philippines and Australia.

Glycosmis arborea (Roxb.) DC. syn *Limonia pentahylla* Retz.. Glabrescent shrubs. Leaves 3-5-foliolate, leaflets oblong-lancelate, up to 10 X 5 cm. Flowers white. Ovary covered with mammillary galnds,5-locular. Berry subglobose, glandular-mammillate, upto 0.5 cm. across.

India, Burma. Frequent across the Ghats, Karnataka, Plant flowring in October to January.

Glycosmis pentaphylla Correa syns. *Limonia pentaphylla* Retz., *Glycosmis chylocaros* W. & A. *Glycosmis arborea* (Roxb.) DC.

Plant occurring in many parts of the area under Upper Gangetic Planis and adjacent Siwaliks and Himalayan tracts; Oudh forests, especially in Dehradun area, and along the base of the Himalaya eastwards, often forming a thick undergrowth.

Glycosmis montana Pierrs.

A small tree in Cochin-China, may possibly be found in Upper Burma, paniclas very short, stamens unequal 5 shorter, anthers not apiculate, style fleshy, as long as ovary. Small tree of 20 ft. height in evergreen forests (species probbaly new). In evergreen forests in Pudaw, Upper Burma, the plant with leaflets 7-9, panicle terminal, large spreading petals rusty-pilose outside; filaments thick, the epipetalous almost sessile.

Some other species of *Glycosmis* Corr. may be indicated :-

Glycosmis mauritiana var. *latifolia* (Kurz.) Balakr.

Glycosmis trifoliata var. *latifolia* Kurz.

G. pentamphylla var. *lattifolia* (Kurz.) Narayan.

Glycosmia macrocarpa W.

Glycosmis pentaphylla var. *macrocarpa* (W.) Hook. f.

Glycosmis longifolia (Hook. f.) Tanaka

Glycosmis pentaphylla var. 2, subvar. *longifolia* Hook. f.

Glycosmis rigida (Jack) Merrill

Glycosmis pentaphylla suvar. *macroplhylla* Hook. f.

Glycosmis angustifolia Lindl.

Glycosmis pentaphylla var. *angustifolia* (Linal. ex. W. & A.)

Glycosmis cymosa (Kurz.) Narayan.

Glycosmis cyanocarpa var. *cymosa* Kurz.

Glycosmis cymosa var. **linearifoliolis** (Tanaka) Mitr. & Subr.

Glycosmis cynanocarpa var. *linearifoliolis* Tanaka

Genus *Glycosmis* Correa in the family Rutaceae (a large family widely distributed over the warmer parts of the world) with salient features - Unarmed shruts or trees. Leaves 1-foliolate or imparipinnate; leaflets alternate. Flowers small, bisexual, in axillary rarely terminal panicles. Calyx 4-5 partite; segments 8-10, broad, imbricate. Petals 4-5, imbricate. Stamens dilated; anthers small often with a dorsal or apical gland. Ovary 2-5-celled; style very short, persistent; stigmas simple; ovules solitary and peduncles in each cell. Berry small, 1-3-seeded. Seeds oblong, testa membranous.

Genus *Glycosmis* Correa has about 6 species, Asiatic and Australian, Species 6 in the Indo-Malayan region.

In family Rutaceae, the genus *Glycosmis* Corx. is among the genera comprising unarmed plants broadly. it is with leaves 3-many-foliolate, leaflets pinnate, flowers bisexual; leaves odd-painnate; leaflets not glaucous beneath and fruit a berry. Anthers glandular and style persistent specifically in *Glycosmis* Corr. plants. The genus is distinguishable from *Murraya* Linn. and *Clausena* N. Burm. having eglandular anthers and style deciduous, and other characters of plants. *Chloroxylon* A.P. de Candolle is also distinguishable for leaves even-pinnate, leaflets glaucous beneath and fruits capsular.

Two species of genus *Glycosmis* Correa are distinguished on the basis of flower characters. Inflorescence equalling or longer than leaf rachis, and ovary ovoid, assile and leaflets crenate in *Glycosmis arborea* (Roxb.) DC; whereas the inflorescence short, ovary fusiform, stalked, leaflets entire and fruit glandular-pitted in *Glycosmis mauritiana* (Lam.) Tanaka.

The roots, fruits, bark and plant of *Gloycosmis* species are medicinally useful.

The roots of *Glycosmis pentaphylla* correa syn. *Glycosmis cochinchinensis* Plierre ex Engler are medicinally used.

Roots are pounded and mixed with sugar and mixture is given in cases of low fever.

Woods are considered useful in snake bite.

Plant contains glycosmin, an active constitutent, identical with veratroylsalicin.

The plant *Glycsmis arborea* (Roxb.) Dc. syn. *G. pentaphylla* Corr. is considered anti-cancer medicine.

Fruits are used in dysentery.

Roots are given in fever as antipyretic medicine. Roots are useful in snake bite. Roots are considered helpful for labour pain in delivery cases. Roots are used in abdominal worms.

Bark is useful in gastric disorders, jaundice and anaemia.

Plant is also considered to be useful in warding off evil spirits in human beings.

Fruits are edible in ripen stage.

The plant *Glycosmis mauritiana* (Lamk.) Tanaka is used medicinally in various diseases.

Fruits are considered useful in throat cancer.

Roots are ground and made into a paste which is applied to wounds and sores.

Roots are used in cough, cold, fever and catarrhal affections

Fruits in ripen state are edible.

Twigs are used as tooth-brush and considered also as a dentrifice

The plant *Glycosmis pentaphylla* Correa syn. *G. arborea* DC. is used in medicine in various ailments. Plant is used in cough, rheumatism, anaemia and jauandice.

The bitter leaves-juice is used in fevers, liver complaints and in worms affection as a vermifuge.

A paste made of leaves and ginger is applied to eczema and skin affections.

The decoction of roots is given for facial inflammations.

The phytochemical screening finds that the air-dried plant material yields two furoquinoline bases, kokusaginine and skimmianine. Other alkaloids found in the leaves are glycosin, arborine, glycosminine and arborinine. Arborine is the major alkaloid of the leaves also existing in the root bark and stem but not in buds, flowers, green fruits and seeds.

Arborine and arborinine isolated from the leaves in yields of 0.5% and 0.12% respectively.

A new alkaloid, glycosine, two netural triterone arborinols A and B. stigmasterol and myricyl isolated from the leaves.

Three new alkaloids glycosamine, glycorine and glycosmicine, as also Y-fagrine and skimmianine isolated from the leaves, while B-sitosterol from the neutral fraction.

Pharmacological ation of alkaloid has been studied. Minor alkaloids glycosmicine, glycorine and glycosmine, and their structure are also observed.

Arbinol, a new triterpene, and isoarbinol from the leaves has been isolated. Two isomeric triterpene alcohols along with myricyl alcohol, stigmasterol and B-sitosterol have also been isolated.

Arborine and arborinine have been isolated from the leaves of *Glycosmis arborea.* Arborine, the major alkaloid, m.p. 155-156° was opitically inactive and had the molecular formula with one N-methyl group. On Soda lime distillation, it gave toluene methylaniline and ammonia.

A critical study of the UV and IR absorption spectra of arborine, it has been shown that arborine is 2-methyl-quinazol-4-one and not the tautameric from 2-bezylidene-1-quinazol-4-one. This was further confirmed by NMR spectrum of arborine.

An alkaloid arhorinine, m.p. 175-176° isolated from the leaves of *Glycosmis arborea* has been found to be optically inactive and has the molecular formula. It has two methoxy groups in addition to one-N-methyl groups and one active hydrogen, present in a hydroxy group. Its structure as established as 2,3-dimethoxy-1-hydroxy-10-methylacaridone.

A minor alkaloid, a-fragrine, m.p. 141-142°, isolated from the plant *Glycosmis arborea*, and 3 other quinazolone derivatives. They are glycosminine, mpp. 270-271°, 1-methyl-2-4-quinazolinedione and glycorine (hygroscopic), m..p. 145-147°, 1-methyl-2-quinazolone, Glycorine, reported as a new 4-quinelone base was found to be skimmianine. The biogenesis of quinazoline has also been provided.

Two isomeric triterpene alcohols of a new type viz. arborinol m.p. 274° and iscarborinol, m.p. 298-99°, from the natural fraction of the light petroleum exttract of *Glycosmis arborea*, alongwith myriol alcohol, m.p 89-90°, stigmasterol and B-sitosterol were isolated. Molecular formulae for both arborinol and isoarborinol were revised.

Methylation and demethylation of the quinazoline alkaloids from *Glycosmis arborea* have also been studied.

Glycozoline, m.p. 181-182°, an optically inactive netural compound having the molecular formula, was isolated from *Glycosmis pentaphylla*. The homogenity of the compound has been esablished by paper and thin layer chromatography. It gave a picrate molecular formula, m.p. 182°. It has one methoxyl and one C-methyl group. The data led to the formulation of glycozoline as 3-methyl-6-methoxy carbazole. The structure has been confirmed by its synthesis.

The strucutre of glycozoline, a carbozole derivative from the root bark of *Glycosmis pentaphylla,* has been shown to be 3-methyl-6-methoxy carbazole.

The isolation of skimmianine and three new acridone alkaloids from the root bark of *Glycosmis pentaphylla* has been made. They were shown to tbe hitherto naturally unknown compounds, based on the spects al finding and chemial correlations; these are noracronycine, m.p. 200°, des-N. methyl-acronycine, m.p. 268-270°, and des-N-methylnoracrony-cine, m.p. 246°. Regarding these compounds, the two possible structures 1-methylxy-2', 2', 10-trimethylpyrano-acridone for acronycine, were found to be more correct.

Pharmacological studies find that the alcoholic extract of the aerial parts of *Glycosmis mauritiana* was found to have CNS depresant activity in mice. The extract produced hypothermia in mice and also reduced amphetsmine hyperactivity.

Arbortine, caused inhibition of the action of acetylcholine on rat uterus, guineapig ileum as well as on skeletal muscle.

Glycosine, an alkaloid from *Glycosmis pentaphylla,* blocked the central action of meascaline and counteracted chemo-convulsions induced by strychnine or metrazol in mice. It also plotentiated the thiopental-induced macrosis and prevented the precipitation of circling movements and convulsions caused by cocaine. The alkaloid also inhbited the contraction of toad's heart and produced hypotension in cats. Its potential utility as a therapeutic agent in some psychomotor disorders has been found.

The screening of biological activity, chemical analysis and isolation of various alkaloids and pharmacological evaluation of *Glycosmis* species provide information on their different aspects.

Medicinal preperties and action of plant drug - Rasa tikta-kaṣāya, madhura (pakva phala), Vīrya uṣṇa, Vipāka kaṭu; Tridoṣa sāmaka (vātakapha hara - pitta saṁsamana); Karma jvaraghna, tvacya, kāsaghna, raktaprssādana, nāḍībalya, dantya, saṅgrāhi, stambhana, sothahara, kaṇṭhya, viṣaghna, krimighna, vraṇa sodhana-ropaṇa, balya, rakṣoghna-bhūtaghna, ākṣephara, pācana and dīpana.

Therapeutic indication in kāsa, jvara, pratisyāya, kaṇṭha-vikāra, āmāsaya-āntra vikāra, atisāRa, pravāhikā, agnimāandya, pānduā kāmalā, vakṛdvikāra-plīhāroga, vrana, carmavikāra, karkatārbuda, haṣṭapraava, sarpadaṁsa, nāḍīrogsa, vatavyadhi, āmavāta, sotha, kṛmiroga, dantavikāra, bhūtavādhā and similar other diseases.

Khādya - phala (pakva).

Vanya Nimbūka, the Sanskrit name for the plant drug.

9

Morinda citrifolia Linn.

Family : Rubiaceae

Regional names : Al, Ach, Surangi, Bartundi (Hindi, Bengla, Gujarati, Marathi), Maddi Togaru (Telugu) Nuna, Tpgaru (Tamil), Ainshi, Tagase, Mad (Kannara), Kattapitalavam, Mannanatti (Malayalam), Achu, Pindra (Oriya), Al (Bombay), Vellainuna (Tamil), Mulugu (Telgu); Chily Ach.

Large shrub or small tree, glabrous. Leaves shining, elliptic blade 6-10 narrowed into pet. 1/2, - 3/4 in. long, stipules large, broadly oblong or semilunar, often 2-3 fid. Peduncles .5 - 1.5 in. usually, solitary, leaf - opposed, the supporting leaf not developed. Flowers 5-merous, corolla-tube up to half inch long. Fruits of many drupes coalescent into fleshy head, pale greeniah-white, 1 in. diam.

Distribution: Darzeeling, Tarai and outer hills, Andamans, as well as along the coast of the Konkan, quite near the sea. Cultivated largely in India and Burma. China, Formosa.

Flowering and fruiting: Autumn or various seasons.

Morinda citrifolia Linn. A small tree with a straight trunk, formerly cultivated throughout the greater part of India and now found only in wild state or as an escape in part of Bengal, Bihar, Orissa, west coast and Andaman Islands.

Small tree with leaves broadly-elliptic, bright green, glabrous; flowers white, in dense ovoid heads; fruits ovoid, glossy, white when ripe; pyrenes compressed, winged on edges.

Morinda pubescens Sm.

Morinda tomentosa roth.

M. tinctoris Roxb.

M. citrifolia Bedd.

M. exerta roxb.

M. leintha Kurz.

M. coreia Buch-Ham.

Family : Rubiaceae

Regional names : Al, Ach (Hindi), Maddi, Togara (Telgu), Nlase (Burma), Ach (Bombay), Manjanatti (Tamil), Rattapiluasum (Malayalam); Achchu, Manjanthi, Podophul.

Small or medium-sized tree, usually pubescent or tomentose. Bark spongy, deeply cracked, greyish-yellow. Leaves not shining, elliptic-obvoate or lanceolatè, blode 4-8, narrowed into petiole about 1/4 in. long. Peduncles solitary, axillary or leaf-opposed, frequently in short trichomous paincles at the ends of branchlets. Flowers scented, 5-merous, corolla usually tomentose outside, tube 1/2-3/4 in. long, anthers exserted or included. Syncarpium 3/4 in. diam.

Flowring and fruiting : July - October or around; March-June

Distribution : Bihar, Central Provinces, Peninsule, Burma, Upper and Lower; often in gardens. Frequently cultivated.

Morinda tinctoria Roxb.

M. tinetoria var. *tomentosa Hook. f.*

M. tinctoria forma *exserta* Gamble

M. exserta Roxb. (in part)

Small tree with 4-angled tomentose branches. Leaves 4-8 in. long. broadly or narrowly elliptic, acute at both ends, tomentose on both surfaces, and shining; petioles short, densely tomentose; stipules often bifid, with narrow acute lobes. Peduncles leaf-opposed or occasionally in axils of a reduced leaf, tomentose. Flowers in globose heads, 5-merous, white. Calyx 1/2 in. long, truncate.

Corolla-tube, aboutt 1 in. long, hairy outside; lobes oblong, obtuse or subacute. Fruits about 1 in. in diam., composed of many coalscent drupes.

Plant occurring in Bengal, Central Provinces and in the Bombay Presidency; probably wild in the forests of various parts of Upper Gangetic Plains, Bundelkhand, also cultivated in the areas; Madhya Pradesh, Uttar Pradesh. Plant flowering during the hot season.

Morinda coreia Buch-Ham. A small tree with fruits 1.3 cm. long glacous green with polygonal marks. Occasional throughout the areas in Madhya Bharat, Madhya Pradesh; Central India. Plant fruits in October.

Morindu tomentosa Heyne ex Roth. syns. iM. tinctoria var. *tomentosa* (Roth.) J. Hooker; *M. tinctoria* Roxb. Shrubby trees. Stipules bifid. Leaves elliptic-lanceolate, acuminate, up to 15 x 6 cm. hairy. Corolla white; tube up to 2.5 cm. long, sparsely hairy. Syncarpium 2 cm. across.

Indomalaysia. Southern India,. Karnataka. Plant flowering and fruiting in March to September.

Morinda tomentosa Hyne., a softly tomentose form. *Morinda angustifolia* Roxb. with distribution in Sikkim-Terai, Burma, lower hills,' assam, Khasi hills, Upper Burma, Pegu (wild and planted by Karena), Tennasserin, Malay Peninsula. A large glabrous shrub; leaves thinly membranous, lanceolate, blade, 4-12 narrowed into petiole short; flowers numerous, fragrant, peduncles axillary or leaf-opposed, corolla, glabrous drupes free. Morinda pernicaefolia Ham. A low shrub or under-shurb; leaves oblanceolate or linear, stipules subulate, peduncles short, leaf-opposed, drupes coalescent.

Morinda angustifolia Roxb.

Regional names : Asho, Darhharidra (Bengla), barr-hardi Huldi-kung (Lepcha), Ashu-goch (Assam), Dieng-nong (Khasi), Chhennong (Gasre), Kawnpel (Lushai), Dieng-seroi (Khasi).

A shurb or small tre found in Eastern Himalayas, Assam, Bihar, Orissa and Andhra Pradesh up to an altitude of 1,800 meters. Leaves large, elliptic or obovate lancolate; flower white and fragrant.

Morinda umbellata Linn. (in part)

Large climbing shrub, climbing by long slender branches, inter-nodes long; leaves usually glabrous and lanceolate, blade 2-5, petiole slender, short or 1/4 in. long; flower heads in terminal sessile umbels, peduncles, 5-10 glabrous or tomentose; up to i in. long, corolla almost rotate throat bearded; syncarpium 1/4 in. diam, irregualrly lobed.

A diffuse or climbing shrub found in Khasi hills, Bihar and Deccan Peninsula at an altitude of 1,500 meters. Leaves elliptic, oblong or lanceolate; flower-heads in terminal sessile umbels and fruit carlet, lobed.

Plant found in west side of the Peninsula in evergreen forests from Coorg-southwards, Khasi hills, Tenasserim, Malay Peninsula, Ceylon moist region to 4,000 ft., common; China, and other regions.

Morinda villous Hook. f. A climbing shrub, branchlets, undersides of leaves and peduncles tomentose. Leaves obovate-elliptic, acuminate, 4-5 in. long secondary nerves 10-15 pair, prominent beneath. Flower heads in terminal umbels, drupes confluent.

Plant occurring in Khasi hills, north-eastern region, India.

Morinda brascteria Roxb. syn. *M. citrifolia* var. *brascteata* Hook. f. A shrub or a small tree found in the coastal forests of Bengal and Deccan Peninsula.

Morinda tomentosa Hyne ex roth. syn. M. tinctoria var. *tomentosa* Hook. fl. A small tree found throughout the greater part of North India and Deccan Peninsula.

Marinds coreia Buch-Ham. has been sometimes censidered as the wild form or a variant of *M. citrifolia* Linn. It is generally known by the same regional or veracular names and put to similar utility.

Besides *Moridna pubescence* Sm. and *M. tinctoria* Roxb. are sometimes treated distinct taxa.

Genus *Marinda* Linn. in the family Rubiaceae (about 500 genera with over 6,000 species; mostly tropical, some temperate and a few Arctic) with salient features - Erect or climbing shrubs or trees, stipules connate, sheathing. Flowers white, sessile on a globose receptacle, the calyces more or less connate, forming dense peduncled flower-heads which are solitary or arranged in panicles or umbles. Calyx limb short, trunclate. Corolla-lobes 4-7, coriaceous, valvate in bud. Stamens 4-7. Ovary 2-or by the prolongation or the placentas spuriously 4-celled, style slender, with 2-stigmate lobes. Fruit as a rule formed of the succulent coalescing drupes, enclosing many cartilaginous or bony 1-seeded pyrenes, which sometimes cohere, drupes rarely free.

Genus *Morinda* in family Rubiaceae (about 76 genera and 274 species in India) has 40 species in tropics of both hemispheres.

The genus belongs to the group of genera with ovules solitary in each cells and corolla-lobes valvate in bud, and leaves not whorled, stipulate; and Morinda is specifically with fruits indehiscent, formed of the succulent, enlarged calyces enclosing many 1-seeded pyrenss, and tree habit.

In family Rubiaceae, the genus *Morinda* Linn. is in tthe tribe Morindeae which commonly have ovules solitary, radicle inferior, corolla-lobes valvate and fruit a drupe or berry. Among the genera of Morindeae such as *Rannellia, Damnacanthus, Gyochthoides* and some others, the genus *Morinda* Linn. is distinguished for the many-fid heads and coehering calyx-lobes; whereas flowers free and ovary 2- or 4-celled in other foregoing genera (two latter) and former is with heads few-fid, fls., violet, calyx limb 4-toothed, when flowers 1 in dense heads, heads many-fid, fls. white and calyx-lobes truncate in *Morinda* Linn., besides other differing characters from other genera of the group.

A group of genera with inflorescence a head and plants trees or shrubs includes *Morinda* Linn. which is distinguished of shurb. or small tree habit and particualrly having calyx-tubes nearly connate and fruits syncarpium; whereas genus *Adina* Salisbury plants are trees with calyx-tubes free and fruit not a syncarpium.

The species of *Morinda* are broadly distinguishable. Corolla 5-7 merous and tube 1/4 in. or longer in *Morinda citrifolia* Linn. and *M. tinctoria* Roxb. ; whereas corolla 4-rarely 5-merous and tubes less than 1/4 in. long. in others, such as Morinda umbellata Linn.

The leaves, bark, fruit and plant *Morinda citrifolia* L. are medicinally useful.

Roots are used as cathartic.

The juice of leaves is auplied exetrnally to gout. Leaves are administered internally as tonic. They are useful as febrifuge in fever. Leaves are applied as paste to wounds and ulcers.

The baked fruits are useful in asthma and dysentery. They are emmenagogue and useful in menstrual troubles.

Unripe berries are charred and mixed with salt applied to spongy gums effectively.

Roots contain glud. morindin; and yeild anthraquinone derivatives.

Specially components of the heartwood from plant are phyto-chemically studied. Roots extractives are found hypotensive and anticongestive. The hypotensor activity of residues in water solution water solvent fraction of the roots.

Special components from the heartwood of plant *Marinda tinctoria* Roxb. are chemically screened.

Woods of the plant contain glycoside morindin.

The roots of the plant Morinda tinctoria Roxb. as well as the bark, fruits, woods and leaves are medicinally useful.

The roots of the plant are exernally applied as well-ground paste to wounds and ulcers.

Plant is useful in fevers in small pox.

The bark is useful in urinary complaints.

Fruits are as bird lime.

The roots, leaves and plant *Morinda angustifolia* Roxb. are medicianlly useful.

The leaves are applied as paste or in the form of juice to sores on feet.

Leaves are useful in giddiness.

The fruits, leaves and roots of the plant *Morinda umbellata* L. are medicinally useful.

Fruits are edible and used in preparation of curry.

Roots of *Morinda angustifolia* Roxb. yield dye. Roots of *Morinda pubescence* Sm. yield yellow dye and the woods are of timber uses.

Various parts of plant *Morinda citrifolia* L. are used medicinally.

The leaves are aplied to cuts and wounds; and the stem bark is also useful in wounds, ulcers and similar ailments.

Leaves are useful in diarrhoea. Leaves are used in fever.

Fruits are used in gum troubles.

The leaves ad stem bark are useful in small pox.

Plant is considered stomachic ad useful in stomach troubles.

Leaves are useful as tonic, and useful in general debility.

Leaves are also edible for use as vegetable.

The fruits of plant *Marinda umbellata* Linn. are edible. Green fruits are used in currles. A decoction of roots and leaves is considered useful in diarrhoea and dysentery.

Root bark contains the colouring principles, mornindone and mornidin. It contains, in addition, a considerable amount of rubichloric acid and small quantities of a trihydroxymethyl anthraquinone methyl ether (m.p. 216°), morindangrin (m.p. 210°), 1.3-dihydroxy 6-methyl anthraquinone (m.p. ·269°), a derivative or dimethyl anthraquinone (m.p. 258°) and a hydroxy -methyl anthraquinone carboxylic acid.

The roots of the plant *Morinda bracteata* Roxb. are of former use in dyeing.

The root of the plant *Morinda tomentosa* Hyne. yields the Al dye. The fruits are eaten. The wood is used for making plates and dishes.

The roots of many of the species of *Morinda* genus were ast one time used in various parts of India for dyeing cotton and also wood and silk, these under the names prevalent in different regions, identified as *Morinda bracteata, M. tomentosa* and *M. coreia* are considered to be the chief source of the dye; and some of the other species of the genus, particualrly, *Morinda braceata, M. tomentosa* and *M. umbellata* were also exploited for the same purpose. Earlier it was considered that most of these dye yielding species as more forms of the very variable *M. citrifolia.*

Plants of *Morinda* species are included in the major source of dye from vegetable origin. In addition some species are of various economic uses, and besides a few species parts is edible and vegetable items.

The roots of *Morinda angustifolia* Roxb. yield a yellow dye, which was foremerly used for dying cotton yarn and clothes; and red shades are obtained on mordanted yarn by using cold water extracts of the roots.

Morinda citrifolia was formerly cultivated as a field crops on an extensive scale and its roots exploited as the source of dye. In cultivation normally, the plant begins to flower and fruit within 2-3 years of planting. After the attaining the age of 3-4 years, the roots are dug out, dried and sorted for use by the dyeing trade. The colouring matter residues in the roots bark and is present to the maximum extent in the plants of 3-4 years age. Best results are obtained from a neutral dye-bath of washed morinda root. Red, purple and chocolate shades are produced on mordanted cotton, silk or wool, the shades being fast to soap. The dyeing powder of morinda root, when necessary precautions are taken, excels that of madder. The use of Al dye has been virtually abondoned since the advent of synthetic dyestuffs.

The colouring principle of morrinda root of *Morinda citrifolia* is morindone (trihydroxy methylanthraquinone) present in the bark mainly as the glucoside morindin; on hydrolysis morindin yields glucose, rhamnose, chloric acid, alizarn, a-methyl ether, rabiadin 1-methyl ether, two isomeric dihydroxy methylanthraquinones (morindadiol and soranjidol) and two trihydroxy methylanthraquinone mono methyl ethers. Morindone may conventionally be prepared in quantity by extacting the roots with sulphurous acid; the non-tinctorial yellow compounds are obtained as by-products; the mcrindone has been synthesized. The woody part mostly contains yellow colouring principles.

Tender leaves of tree *M. citrifolia*, grown as shade tree and support for pepper vines, are eaten. Trees are lopped for fodder and the leaves are used to rear silkworms. The pulp of the fruits is used for cleansing hairs.

The fruits yield a small amount of yellow essential oil (specific gravity 0.927) consisting mainly of hexoic and octoic acids with small quantities of a paraffin (m.p. 60°) and esters of ethyl and methyl alcohols. The wood of the tree is yellowsih brown, fairly hard and close-grained.

Many parts of the plant are considered to possess medicinal properties; and the roots, fruits and leaves are mainly used in various ailments externally and internally.

The tree of *Morinda coreia* is lopped for fodder. Analysis of leaves finds the values - nitrogen 2-02, calcium 3-77, and ash 9.33%. The roots of the plant were formerly used in dyeing cotton. The wood is light red when freshly cut, often with yellow streaks, chaging in dull red with age. It is smooth, somewhat lustrous, straight - grained, medium - textured, moderately hard to hard and light. Woods are used for making several items of use as economic utility.

The root bark contains morindone and its glucoside morindin. Heasrtwood contains three anthraquinone pigments, namely morindone, damnacanthal and nordamnacanthal.

Medicinal properties and action of plant drug - Raa ttikta-kaṣāya, vīraya-uṣṇa, Vipāka kaṭu; Tridaṣasāmaka; and Karma jvaraghna, grāhi, stambhana, balya, vraṇaropaṇa-spdhana, kāsaghna, svāsahara, vedanāsthāpana, dantya, dantamūla-sothahara, sothahara, mūtrala and dīpana.

Therapeutic indication for internal and external uses in Jvara, dantamūlasotha, pradara, atisāra, pravāhikā, vrana, kāsa, svāsa, sandhisotha, daurbalya, masūRikā, mūtraroga and ārtavaikāra, and other ailments.

Khādya - phala, sāka tathā āhāra - vyañjana

Ārthika upayogitā - rañgadravya; tathā vividha

Rañjanamūlā, the Sanskrit name for the plant drug.

10

Naregamia alata W. & A.

Turrea alata wight W. & A. *Naregamia dentata* Miq.

Family : Meliaceae

Regional names: Pittvel, Pittapapra, Pittmari, Tinpini (Marathi), nela-neringu, nala-kanu-gida (Kannarese), Nela-meragam (Malayalam), Trifolio (Goa); Nilanarai.

Small glabrous undershrub. Branches erect or decumbent, from a few inches to 2 ft. long. Leaves 1-4 in. long; terminal leaflets rather larger than the lateral ones and about the length of the common petiole. Flowers 1-1.5 in. long, quite white, longer than the peduncles. Style yellow.

Flowering and fruiting : Summers and other seasons.

Distribution : Western Peninsula, or the Western Ghas from the Concan southwards. Angola (a pubescent form).

Naregamia alata W. & A. A shining undershrub and small glabrous undershrub, with leaflets sessile, cuneate-obovate quite entire or obtusely lobed, common petioles winged.

Plant occurring in Southern India; Konkan, West Kanara, Western of Madras State upto 3,000 ft. in various districts.

Genus *naregamia* W. & A. in the family Meliaceae (about 300 species, mostly tropical, widely spread over both hemispheres, and near about 113 species in Indian Archipelago), with salient features. Small glabrous and shining undershrub. Leaves trifoliolate. Peduncles axillary, solitary, 1-flowered.

Calyx small, campanulate, 5-cleft, deciduous. Petals 5, free, elongate-spathulate, imbricated in bud, at length spreading above. Staminal-tube elongated, inflated above, obsoletely 10-crenate at the mouth, exerted, setaceous-apiculate. Disk annular. Ovary 3-celled, evoues 2 collateral in each cells, pendulous; style filiform, stigmas capitate. Capsules ovoid-globose, 2-lobed, 3-celled, loculicidally 3-valved; valves separating from the 3-winged axis. Seeds 2 in each cells, albumen fleshy; embryo foliaceous.

Genus *Naregamia* in Tribe Melieae (in family Meliaceae) with main features-leaflets ofen toothed. Stamens united into a tube. Cells of ovary 1-2-ovuled. Seeds not winged, albumen thin fleshy; cotyledons thin, foliaceous. Genus *Naregamia* belongs to group of genera with plants having trifoliolate pinnate or 2-3 pinnate, such as in *Melia* Linn. (tree), *Murronia* Wight. (shrubs or undershrubs) and *Cipadessa* Blume (shrubs or small trees); when single genus *Turreae* Linn. in this tribe has simple leaves. Specifically the genus *Naregamia* W. & A. has winged petiole and ovule collateral, which carries distinction in comparison to other genera like *Murronia* Wight. and *Melia* Linn. with petioles not winged and ovules apressed (and these two genera further differ the character of disk, petals and fruit mutually). These genera have common characters of elongated flowers and style long, the genus *Naregamia* W & A. is distinguishable for characteristics of flowers, leaves-petiole, ovules and petals - flowers and other salient features. Genus *Cipadessa* Blume. is separated of flowers globose and styles rather short and some other characters.

The roots, leasves, stems and plant of *Naregamia alata* Wt. & Arn. are medicinally useful.

The roots are useful in inflammation of naval region.

Roots are emetic , cholagogue, expectorant and useful in acute dysentery.

Leaves and stems are useful in decoction administration with bitters and aromatics in biliousness.

Plant is used in rheumatism and itch.

Root bark contains alkaloid naregamin.

Medicinal properties and action of the plant drug - Rasa kaṭu - tikta-kaṣāya, Vīrya uṣṇa, Vipāka kaṭu; Vatakaphahara-pittasamsamana; and Karma Vāmaka, pittavīrecaka, sothahara, āmapācana, kaphanihsāraka, kaṇḍūghna, vedanāsthāpana and tvacya.

Theraputic indication in āmavāta, kāsa, svāsa, pravāhikā, pittavikāra, kaṇḍu., nābhisotha and other ailments.

This plant drug consists of the creeping roots and the slender stems attached to them. The roots have pungent aromatic odour. The effect of the roots as emetic and expectorant with action similar to those obtained from the drug Ipecauanha, given in equal doses.

The other extract contains an alkaloid, an oxidisable and fixed oil and a wax.

In dysentery the decoction of bark in rice water is used and considered curing medicine. In Goanese, the name Avacari means to emetic, and name Trifolia is a version of Marathi name Tinpini.

Pītikā, the Sanskrit name for the plant drug.

11

Phlogacanthus thyrasiformis (Hard) Mabb.

Phlogacanthus thyrasiflorus (Roxb.) Nees.

Justicia thyrsiflora Roxb.

Justicia thyrsiformis Hard.

Family : Acanthaceae

Regional names : Bakhatita (Assameae-Begla), Lal-bahuk (Punjabi), Kaidona (Garhwal); jabuit, Jiamerymbur, Kising, Nokam, Titaphul.

Erect, perennial undershrubs. Stems 4-gonous, thickened, often purple-tinged on the nodes. Leaves drooping, on 1-1.5 cm. long petioles, oblanceolate - oblong to elliptic, attenuate towards the base, acuminate, glabrous, glossy and dark green above, 8-25 X 4-6 cm. Flowers in 4 to 5-0.2-0.25 cm. longs. Bracts 3, linear-subulate; other ones 0.5-0.7 cm. long. Calyx-segments linear-setaceous, villous, 1 cm. long. Corolla brick-red, 1-1.3 cm. long. Caplsule glabrous.

Flowering and fruiting : March - April : May June

Distribution : Subtropical Himalayas upto 4,600 ft. from Ravi to Bhutan, also in Assam. Chota Nagpur and extending to Upper and Lower Burma.

Phlogacanthus thyrsiflorus Nees.

Evergreen shrub, up to 8 ft. high, with smooth grey bark; shoots swollen at the nodes, often fringed with dull purple,

4-angled. Leaves drooping 6-8 in. long, elliptic-lanceolate, obtuse subentire, dark green and glossy above, paler beneath and densely punctuate, petioles up to 1 in. long.

Flowers pedicelled, crowded in verticals of four, forming terminal elongate thyrsoid panicles up to 12 in. long; bracts subulate, conspicuous in bud, arranged in threes, the 2 inner ones persistent; the outer larger caducous. Calyx-segments bristle-like, hairy. Corolla orange-coloured or brick-red, villous, tube laterally compressed; upper lip suberect, deeply emarginate; lower spreading, of 3 ovate acute lobes. Anthers dark-brown, pollen white. Capsule small, linear-clavate, glabrous. Seeds 12-14, densely hairy.

Plant occurring commonly in moist shady places in forests of foothills, terai and Siwalik range, and esastwards in the sub-Himalayan tracts of Rohilkhand and North Oudh; the Upper Gangetic Plains.

Phlogacanthus thyrsiflorus Nees. A semi-evergreen shrub, bark pale - brown, slightly rough. Twigs pale, often whitish with large pith. Young shoots quadrangular and narrowly winged. Leaves oblanceclate, entire, acuminate, usually caudate, base cuneate, glabrous, dark glossy green above, pale glaucescent beneath, lateral nerves 8-12 pairs. Flowers orange red in dense spikelike, densely pubescent panicles; spikes terminal, usually solitary. Pedicel and calyx clothed outside with purplish brown pubescent. Filament yellow. Anthers purple. Capsule sub-quadrangular.

Plant throughout the sub-Himalayan tract and outer ranges ascending to about 100 meters elevation. Plant lower and fruits during the period from spring to summer. Generally plant shows a tendency to spread upwards from areas and elevation of its occurrence.

Phlogacanthus pubinervius T. Anderson.

Family : Acanthaceae

Evergreen hairless shrub up to 3 meters, with 4 - angled grey branches, and with drooping leaves with oblanceolate blades 15-25 cm., narrowed to a stalk. Showy in early spring with its dense cylindrical splikes of brick-red velvety, 2-lipped tubular flowers 8-25 cm. long, and with conspicuous bracts in bud. Corolla broad-tubular, curved, 2-2.5 cm., 2-lipped with 5 nearly equal lobes, stamens exserted; calyx-lobes 6-8 mm. bristly-haried; bracts 6-12 mm. long. .

Capsule cylindrical 4-angled, hairless, up to 4 cm.; seeds disk-like, finely hairy.

Flowering and fruiting February - March and onwards.

Distribution : Uttar Pradesh to Bhutan, Northern India, Burrma; from 200 to 1700 meters elevation firests.

Gymnostachym latifolium (Dalzel) T. Anderson.

Cryptophragmium latifolium Dalzell.

Phlogacanthus latifolius Wight.

Family : Acanthaceae

Undershrubs. Petiole 6-16 cm. long, glaucous when young; blade 12-20 X 12-16 cm., broadly ovate-orbicular, acute at apex, rounded to subcordate at base, glabrous. Inflorescence an axillary panicle of racemes; bracts ovate, acuminate; bracteoles smaller. Calyx lobes ovate, acuminate. Corolla greenish yellow, upto 2 cm. long, glabrous; lobes short, rounded. Stamens 2, exerted. Capsule linear, with compressed with seeds.

Flowering and fruiting : November - April

Distribution : South - West India Common in lower Ghats, along streams in shade of wet deciduous and semi-evergreen forest undergrowth.

Gymnostachyam febrifugum Benth

Gymostachym alatum Wight.

Family : Acanthaceae

Regional names : Nelaumchacala (Kannarese)

Nearly stemless herb. Leasves 6.5 by 3 in., decurrent on the petiole, subentire or undulate - crenulate, above lineolate nearly glabrous or minutely sparsely setulose, beneath paler glabrous or pubescent on the nerves. Panicles 6-12 in. in appearance radical, flowers opposite, solitary or in very small few-fid cymes; bracts small, narrow; bracteoles O. Sepals small, glabrous or puberulous. Corolla glabrous. Anthers ovate, hairy. Capsule 1 in.

Distribution : South Deccan Peninsula; also South Kanara.

Genus *Gymnostachym* Nees in family Aanthaeeae, with salient features. Herbs or undershrubs; stem often thickened above nodes. Leaves sometimes radical. Inflorescence usually axillary, of cymes or panicles of narrow racemes; bracts and bracteoles small. Calyx of 5, small or subequal lobes. Corolla tube widening towards limb, more or less curved; limb bilabiate. Stamens 2, sometimes exserted; staminodes O; anther cells 2, parallel, glabrous or hairy. Ovary sometimes hairy; locules 6-many-ovuled. Capsule linear.

Genus *Gymnostachym* Nees with 15 species, Indian, with a few Malayan, is among the group of species having panicle terminal leafless or nearly so, and particualrly leaves mostly near the base of the stem. *Gymnostachym febrifugum* Bentham. is distinguished from *Gymnostachym latifolium* (Dalzel). A. Anderson by its subradical leaves, and the leaf blade being decurrent on to the petiole and its general habit as a whole.

Various other species of the genus *Gymnostachym* Nees. Nees. have distribution mainly in Southern India, Western

Deccan Peninsula, Karnataka, Khasia hills, Malabar, Concan and Ceylon; also in Central India (*Gymnostachym tomentosum* T. Anders.). Genus *Phlogacantus* Nees. differ from genus Gymnostachym Nees in the broader, curved corolla, the glabrous ovary, and the much stouter capsule, and other features.

Genus *Phlogacanthus* Nees in family Acanthaceae (about 68 genera with over 337 species in India) with salient features - Shrubs or tall herbs. Leaves entire or obscurely crenate. Flowers in terminal thyrses or narrow panicles, rarely in axillary racemes or cymes; bracts small, bracteoles none. Calyx 5-partite segments very narrow. Corolla tubular, curved upwards, tube narrowly funnel - shapped limb more or less 2-lipped; lobes ovate or oblong, connivent spreading or recurved, imbricate in bud. Stamens 2, with sometimes 2 small rudiments added, anthers 2-celled, oblong, muticous, glabrous. Ovary with 508 ovules in each cell, glabrous, style filiform, stigmas subsimple. Fruit an elongated many-seeded capsule, lenticular, ovate in outline, glabrous or densely puberulous.

Genus *Phlogacanthus* Nees is in Tribe 5 Justiciease and Subtribe 1 Androgrophideae with salient characters of ovules 3-10 in each cell and capsule normally 6-or more-seeded, and specifically corolla cylindric, curved not ventricose nor deeply 2-lipped in *Phlogacanthus* Nees, which is characteristic in a group of genera having capsule subterete and seeds much compressed, for the instance, in certain genera like *Gymnestachym* Nees, *Cystacanthus* T. Anders and *Dictanthus* Benth, but these genera differ by characters of corolla mainly. For the example, the corolla ventricose and not deeply 2-lipped in genus *Cystacanthus;* and corolla-tube very slender and limb small in *Gymnostachym,* and corolla deeply 2-lipped in genus *Dictacanthus.* Besides genus *Phlogacanthus* belongs to genera of family having the fertile stamens 2 broadly.

There are thirty Indo-Malesian species and 10 or 11 (10 to 12) splecies in India (endemic in India), all are Himalayan, confined to Eastern Himalaya, with 1 extending to North Himalaya (1,320 meters).

Various species of the genus *Phlogacnthus* Nees. are also separated majorly on the basis of characteres of panicles, as many species are with thyres or dense panicles terminal, and only a few are with cymes or short panicles axillary. (*Phlogacanthus pubinervis* T. Anders and *P. jankisii* Clarke.). Some species falling in former kind of character may be indicated Phlogacanthus curviflorus. Nees., *P. tubiflorus* Nees, *P. phyrisiflorus* t. Anders, *P. guttatus* Nees, *P. elongatus* T. Anders, *P. asperulus* Nees and *P. wallichii* Clarke.

Phlogacanthus guttatus Nees

Family : Acanthaceae

Regional names : Khie-nerymbul

Shrub. Leaves large oblong or elliptic acuminate at both ends glabrous, panicles linear dense somewhat pubescent, calyx-teeth 1/6 in., leaves often 9 by 3 in.; petiole 1.5 in. Panicles 3-6 by 1 in, terminal or quasiterminal, solitary or 2-3 together. Corolla pubescent, 2-lipped, segments oblong patent subrcurved, yellow; upper lip of corolla subercet. lower deeply 3-lobed, green with purple spots. Capsule 12-seeded.

Distribution : Khasia Hills, elevation of 2,00 - 4,000 ft., on the southern face, common.

Phlogacanthus tubiflorus Nees.

Justicia tubiflora Wall.

Family : Acanthaceae

Regional names : Chakbam

Shrub. Leaves 10 by 3-5.5 in., subentire of crenulate, densely punctulate above, almost wooly (but deciduously) pubescent beneath; leaves large elliptic or ovate narrowed at hboth ends softly pubescent beneath; petiole 1-2 in. Panicle 2-8 in., densely closely ramous, subthyrsoid; pedicels often 1/4 in.;' bracts 1/8 in., linear, Calyx-tube 1/18 in.; teeth linear-lanceolate, pubescent or glabrate; calyx-teeth 1/8 in., corolla 3/4 in. tubular curved scarcely widened upwards. Panicle 2-8 in., densely closely ramous, subthyrsoid; Capsule glabrous, 12-seeded. Seeds much compressed, glabrous.

Distribution : Assam Plains and adjacent Khasia Terai, elevation 2,000 ft.

It is closely allied to *Phlogacanthus asperulus* Nees. *guttatus* Nees., but the leaves are larger, the corolla larger and altogether a different shape and colour (of *P. guttatus*). The corolla of *Phologanthus tubiflorus* Nees. is nearly as of *Phlogacanthus wallichii* Clarke. The species is allied to *Phlogacanthus wallichii* Nees. but differing in the softly hairy under surface of the leaves and the much more open panicles.

The flowers, roots, stems, leaves and plant of *Phlogacanthus* species are medicinal useful. Plant *Phlogacanthus thyrsiflours* Nees is medicinally useful as *Adhatods vaica* Nees.

Leaves are useful in bronchitis. Leaves are used in cold and cough. Roots are considered useful in cough and colds. The leaves are useful diarrhoea, dysentery and fever.

Leaves are useful in indigestion and stomach disorders. Roots of the plant are medicinally used in various ailments. The roots are useful in cold, cough and bronchitis.

The stems are useful in diarrhoea and dysentery, and also in fever.

Flowers are edible and used as a vagetable. Leaves are utilised as fodder.

The leaves of *Phlogacanthus guttatus* Nees. are medicianlly useful. Leaves are applied over insect bites.

Whole plant of *Phlogacanthus tubiflorus* Nees, are also possessing importance in religious ceremony.

The roots or whole plant of *Gynostachym febrifugum* Wight. are considered useful in fever.

The medicinal properties and action of plant drug—Rasa Tikta - kaṣāya, Vīrya uṣṇa, Vipāka kaṭu, Guṇa laghu-rūksa; Pittakapha sāmaka; Karma jvaraghna, kasahara, svedajanana, sleṣmanihsāraka, mutrala, stambhana and pacana.

Therapeutic indication in Kāsa, savāsa, jvara, kītadaṁsa, mutrala, stambhana and pacana.

Therapeutic indication in Kāsa, svāsa, jvara, kītadaṁsa, atisāra, pravāhikā, sleṣmavikāra, āmāsayaroga, agnimāndya, daurbalya and other similar ailments.

Khadya - puṣpa, sāka

Pasu cikitsā - patra, pasukhādya

Supuṣpā , the Sanskrit name for plant drug.

12

Stachyrarpheta jamaicensis (L.) Vahl.

Stachytarpheta indica (L.) Vahl.

S. jamaicensis (Linn.) Vahl. var. *indica* H.J. Lam.

S. indica such non Vahl.

Verbena jamaicensis L.

Family : Verbenaceae

Regional names: Simainayuruvi (Marathi), Kariyutarani (Kanarese), Katapunullu (Malayalam); Koraputla, Longri.

Subscandent, sparsely pubescent undershrubs. Leaves similar to that of another allied species (*S. mutabilis*). Spikes up to 30 cm. long. Corolla blue-purple; limb up; to 0.8 cm. across.

Flowering and fruiting : All seasons: August - February

Distribution : Tropical Countries, Tropical America; naturalised in tropical parts of Asia.

Stachytlparphita indica Vahl.

Erect, glabrous undershrub. Leaves ovate to ellipltic, toothd. Flowers blue, pretty, in long, terminal, bracteate spikes. Plant flowering from the rains to spring seasons and fruiting within the period.

Plant occurring frequently across plains, Karnatkaa. Planted in Gardens, northern India, Delhi, Dehradun area and various other areas. From Punjab and Sylhet tc Travancore. Naturalised and cultivated both states.

Stachytarphata indica Vahl. A nearly glabrous herb. 1-2 ft. high. Leaves elliptic serrate. Flowers dark-blue, in long slender termial spikes.

Plant is nattive of South America, but cultivated in many and most tropical countries and subtropical regions, and often occurring as a naturalised wood. Plant frequently found in the areas of Upper Gangetic Plains and Siwaliks ranges.

Plant has natural hydridisation in India.

Stachytarpheta mutabilis (N.Jacq.) Vahl.

Verbena mutabilis N.Jacq.

Family : Verbenaceae

Sparsely white-pubescent undershrubs. Petiole 1-2 cm. long; blade ovate, decurrent along the petiole; blade ovate, decurrent along the petiole. Spike up to 40 cm. long, arched; bracts lanceolate; calyx up to 1.5 cm. long. Corolla pink-red, up to 2 cm. long; limb up to 1.2 cm. across.

Flowering and fruiting : All seasons.
Plant used as hedge and often cultivated.

Distribution : Karnataka state, India.

Another species of genus *Stachylarpheta* Vahl. may be referred :

Stachytarpheta urticaefolia (Shisb.) Sims.

Cymburus urticaefolisu Salisb.

Staschytarpheta indica auct. non Vahl.

Genus *Stachytarpheta* Vahl. in the family Verbenaceae (75 genera and 3,000 species in tropics and subtropics; 17 genera with over 96 species in India) with salient features - Large herbs or shrubs, sometimes subscandent. Leaves dentate. Inflorescence a terminal, centripetal spike. Flowers sessile and subtended by persistent bracts or immersed in the rachis and ebracteate, 4-merous. Calyx tubular, ribbed, dentate. Corolla salverform; tube slightly curved, hairy inside; limb oblique, with spreading, often emarginate lobes. Stamens 2. Staminodes 0-2, linear small. Ovary 2.locular, 2-ovulate; style elongate, persisting; stigmas subcapitiate. Druples included in calyx, breaking into two 1 seeded pyrenes.

Two species of the genus *Stschytarpheta* Vahl. may be distinguishable. Spike villous and 1 cm. across in *Stachytarpheta mutabilis* (N. Jacq.) Vahl.; whereas the style glabrascent 0.5 cm. across in *Stachytarpheta indica* (L.) Vahl.

Genus *Symphorema* Roxb. initially belongs to the genra in Verbenaceae bearing simple leaves, when the genus *Vitex* Linn. has digitately 3-7-foliolate. Broadly the group of genera having herbs, shrubs, or small trees (less than 12 meters), with leaves and inflorescence less than 30 cm. and fruiting calyx only slightly accrescent, include genus Stachytarpheta Vahl. which is specifically with the inflorescence subtended by a whorl of 6, foliaceous, accrescent leaves and staments 6 or more.

Bu Guṇa laghu, rūkṣa; Vātakaphahara (tridoṣa sāmaka); and Karma jvaraghna, sveda-jnana, caksusya, vraṇaropana, krimighna, dīpana-pacana, grāhī, vedanāsthāpana, śothāhara, kāsaghna, garbhasrāvakara, kaṇḍūghna, āmapācana, raktaprsādana and stambh*ana*.

Therapeutic indication in Atisāra, pravāhikā, viṣūcikā, āmadoṣa, agnimāndya, krimiroga, netraroga netāhbhisyanda - timira, kaṇḍū, pāmā, carmavikāra, ratijaroga, jvara, vraṇa, śotha, āmavāta, sindhiśotha, śūla, kāsa, śvāsa, phuphusavikāra, kṣata, tvagdoṣa and śūla.

Suparṇā, the Sanskrit name for plant drug.

The leaves, roots and plant of *Stachytarpheta jamaicensis* (L.) Vahl. are medicinally useful.

Leaves are useful as maturant.

Plant is externally used for purulent ulcers. Plant is nternally given in fevers and for rheumatism, arthritic nflammation. Plant is useful in dysentery.

Plant contains glucosidic substance.

The roots are considered abortifacient. Roots are also useful in pneumonia, and other chest complaints.

The leaves are stomachic, and useful in dysentery and cholera and also similar gastrointestinal troubles.

Leaves are applied to scabies, cuts and wounds, and other skin affections.

Plant is useful in eye diseases particualrly catract and conjunctivitis.

Plant is considered useful in veneral diseases. Plant is used as anthelmintic. It is useful in rheumatism.

Medicinal properties and action of the plant drug - Rasa kaṭu-tikta-kaṣāva, Vīrya uṣṇa, Vipāka kaṭu, Guṇa laghu, rūkṣa; Vātakaphahara (tridoṣa sāmaka); and Karma jvaraghna, sveda-janana, caksusya, vraṇaropana, krimighna, dīpana-pacana, grāhī, vedanāsthāpana, sothahara, kāsaghna, garbhasrāvakara, kaṇḍūghna, āmapācana, raktaprsādana and stambhana.

Therapeutic indication in Atisāra, pravāhikā, viṣūcikā, āṃadoṣa, agnimāndya, krimiroga, netraroga - netrāhbhisyanda - timira, kaṇḍū, pāmā, carmavikāra, ratijaroga, jvara, vraṇa, sotha, āmavāta, sindhisotha, sūla, kāsa, svāsa, phuphusavikāra, kṣata, tvagdoṣa and sūla.

Suparṇā, the Sanskrit name for plant drug.

13

Solena amplexicaulis (Lamk) Gandhi

Solena heterophylla (Lour.) Cgogn.

Melothria heterophylla (hour) Cogn.

Zehneria umbellata (Kien. ex Willd) Thw.

Karivia umbellata

Bryonia filiformis Roxb.

Bryonia emplexicaulis Lem.

Momordica umbellata Roxb.

Family: Cucurbitaceae

Regional names: Tarali, *Amantmul (Hindi), Kudari* (Bengla Bombhur), Thiyyadonda (Telgu), Pulivanji (Tamil),

Njeringanpuli (Malayalam), Karakiya(Ori*esses),* having leaf shape cordate and leaf shape ovate in *Bremna latifolia* which (both) are distinct. having other characters also.

Solena amplexicaulis (Lamk) Gandhi

Solena heterophylla (Lour.) Cgogn.

Melothria heterophylla (hour) Cogn.

Zehneria umbellata (Kien. ex Willd) Thw.

Karivia umbellota

Bryonia filifermis Roxb.

Bryonia amplexicaulis Lem.

Momordica umbellata Roxb.

Family: Cucurbitaceae

Regional names: Tarali, Amantmul (Hindi), Kudari (Bengla Bombhur), Thiyyadonda (Telgu), Pulivanji (Tamil),

Njeringanpuli (Malayalam), Karakiya(Oriesses), Matka, Makirla (Oriya), Comotta (Bombay), Denkakra (Punjab), Bukunduru (Mun dari), Soli-khia-phlang (Khasi), Zongawm pawng (Lushai), Tiddands (Telgu), Gometi (Bombay-Marathi); Bankundri, (Gomati, Gwalkakri, Mahakal, Rakhalsuse, Kval-karkri, Bank karela.

Perennials, Stems sulcate, glabrous. Tendrils simple. Leaves ovate-triangular to sagitate or suborbicular, entire to 3-5 -lobed-partite, denticulate, cordate-sagitate at base, scabrid above, glabrous, smooth, gland-punctate or the lower surface, 4-15x 2-8 cm. Male flower in corymbs. Pedicals 0.8 -1.5 cm. long. Calyx 0.5 cm. long; lobes subulate, Corolla yellowish; segments triangular, glandular-pubescent, 0.13-0.15 (-3 cm.) long. Disk orange-yellow. Female flowers solitary, Pedicels 0.7-0.8 cm. long. Ovary smooth, 3-gonous, ribbed, muricate, densely pubescent. Fruit oblong-ovoid, 3-6 cm. long angular or ribbed.

Flowering and fruiting : March - November

Distribution : Throughout India; from India to Ceylon, also in China, Cochinchina and in Java,

Melothria heterophylla (Lour.) Cogniaux

Scandent herb. Root perennial consisting of several tubers, Stems branched, glabrous. Tendrils simple. Leaves and polymorphous, regularly ovate or 3-5-angled, usually cordate at the base, pale green above, paler and reticulately veined beneath. Male flowers subumbellate, 15-20 on a peduncle, corolla small, yellowish white. Female flowers peduncles solitary. Fruit oblong, ovoid, cylindric, tapering towards the aptex, bright red when ripe.

Plant occurring in various provinces in country ascending up to 2,100 meters in hilly regions, Scandent herb with tuberous roots found in flowering and fruiting states from summers to autumn usually.

Melothria amplexicaulis (am.) Cogn.

Dioecious climbers. Leaves remotely denticulate, ovate, obtuse-acuminate, clasping at base, up to 9 X 5 cm., slightly scabrous,. membranous. Staminate flowers in a short corymbs. Pistillate flowers solitary. Corolla creamy-white. Staminal filsments distinct, glabrous; connective produced. Berry oblong, ribbed 2-3 cm. long.

Plant growing in Southern India. Occasional in western plains and upper Ghats, Karnataka. Herb flowers during the spring to rains or onwards.

Solena heterophylla Cogn.

A perennial climbing herb. Roots tuberous. Tendrils very long. Leaves very variable, ovate, oblong, suborbicular or narrowly lanceolate in outline, entire or variously lobed and sometimes nearly to the base, often cordate or hastate at the base, acute or acuminate, denticulate, rough above, usually smooth beneath, Male fls. corymbose; Calyx glabrous, teeth subulate; corolla yellowish white; Anthers densely ciliate. female fls. solitary on short peduncles. Fruit oblong, cylindric, red (ripen stage). Seeds many, subglobose, not margined, smooth.

Plant found common within the areas under Upper Gangetic plains, adjacent subtropical Himalayas, Siwaliks, Terai and Bhawar areas. Mostly herb occurring below 1200 meters and ascending up to 1800 or 2000 meters in western Himalayas regions, or lower hilly region in northern India.

Solena amplexicaulis (Lamk) Gandhi syn. **Zehneria umbellata** Thwaites. A scandent perennials. Leaves polymorphous, ovate, sub-orbicular, oblong or narrowly lanceolate undivided or variously lobed, remotely denticulate; flowers small, yellow; male flowers various, sub-umbellate, bollate, racemes or densely or laxly fascicled; female flowers solitary. Fruits oblong, brown, red (ripe), with many subpherical, smooth seeds.

Plant common in scrub jungles, forest clearings, forest edges, hedges and sal forests; Siwalik range, Uttar Pradesh

Melothria purpusilla Cogn.

Bryonia hookeriana *&. A.*

Zehneria hookeriana *Arn.*

Melothria cissioides *Wall.*

Family : Cucurbitaceae

Regional names : Bankundri (Hindi)

Herb with very slender stems. Leaves evate, cordnate, entire or angled, rarely 3-5-lobed, acute, mucronate or shortly acuminate, denticulate, scabrous above and usually glabrous beneath; petiols up to 2 in. long. Flowers monoecious, pale-yellow, the males capitate or umbellate at the apex of the common peduncle. Calyx-teeth very short, recurved. Filaments villous, connective, not produced. Female solitary or subumbelled. Fruit globose, small, finely reticulate, glabrous. Seeds small, compressed, distinctly margined, smooth.

Flowering and fruiting : Spring to Autumn seasons

Distribution : Nepal, East Bengal and Eastern Himalyas up to 5,000 ft.; India, Assam, Bengal, South Indi and other regions. Also in Java.

Melothria perpusilla Cogn. A quite slender plant occurring in Upper Gangetic Plains, Central India, Madhya Pradesh,

Uttar Pradesh, Siwalik ranges. Herb in Southern regions of country, Konkan, Deccan, Western Ghats and Karna·aka.

Zehnria maysorensis (Wight. & Arnot.) Arn.

Bryonia maaysorensis Wight & Arn.

Melothria perpusilla var. *subtruncata* Gogn.

Melothria perpusilla acut. non (Blume) Gogn.

Family : Cucurbitaceae

Monoecious climber. Leaves remotely serrate, ovate, suborbicular or oblong, simple to 3-7-lobed, up to 9 X 7 cm., often hispid beneath, membranous. Flowers sub-umbellate or pistillate, flowers solitary subsessile; sometimes stamiate and pistillate flowers coaxillary. Corolla white. Stamens inserted as the base of calyx; filaments pilose. Berry 1 cm. across, smooth with age; seeds smooth, apiculate.

Flowering and fruiting : All seasons

Distribution : Indomalaya. Occassional in undergrowth in wet deciduous forests of upper Ghats.

Zehneria hookeriana Arn.

Climbing herb. Leaves cordate, acute, simple or angular or 5-lobed half-way down, petiole, longer than the auricles. Fruit small, when dry reticulate-rugose globose; seeds much flattened oblong margined smooth or slightly tuberculate on the face.

Plant distirbution in Ava, Malaya, Africa, North Bengal; common in Sikkim, Assam, Khasia hills and Cachar, ascending to 5,000 ft. Deccan Peninsula and Ceylon; common, in the lower hills usually.

Mukia maderaspatana (L.) Roemer

Melothria madrespatana (L.) Cogn.

Cucumis madrespatana L.
Bryonia scabrella L.
Bryonia scabrella L.
Mukia scabrella (Linn. f.) Arn.
Kerivia javanica Miq.
Bryonia wightiana Wall.
Family : Cucurbiataceae
Regional names : Agumuki, Gwal-kakri (Hindi); ankh phod ki bel, Akhphor, Ankhphulini-ki-bel, Gowasi.

Scandent or prostrate annual, with slender angular hispid or scabrous stems. Leaves 1-3 in., in ovate or subdeltoid, entire, angled or 3-5-lobed, acute or subacuminate dentate or coarsely serrate, very rough. Flowers monoeicious, yellow. Male flowers in cluster. Calyx-tube villous; teeth subulate. Corolla hairy outside. Connective of stamens produced. Female flowers axillary or subfascicled. Fruits small, globose, very shortly stalked, bright red when ripe. Seeds turgid.

Flowering and fruiting : July - December
Distribution : Throughout India to Ceylon; also in the Malay Archipelago, Formosa and in Australia.

Mukia scabrella Arn.

Scabrous climbing herb. Stems angualr, slender, hispid or very scarbid. Leaves rough hispid beneath, 1-3 in., serrate; petiole often very short, some times 1 in. or more. Flowers small. Ovary very hisid. Fruit small, bright red. Seeds rough on their faces.

Mukia maderaspatana (L.) Roemer

Scandent or decumbent herb. Leaves serrate, ovate, acute, upto 7 X 6 cm., scabrous. Flowers small. Corolla yellow. Staminal filaments pilose, short; connective apiculate. Berry 1 cm. across, short-pedicelled, red with age.

Plant distribution in Paleotropics. Southern India, Karnataka. Maharashtra. Tamilnadu and other regions.

Mukia maderaspatana (L.) R. syn. *Melothria maderaspatana* Cogn.

Annuals. Stems sulcate, patently hisplid. Tendrils simlple. Leaves broadly ovate-reniform, entire to 3 to 5-angled or -lobed, denticulate-dentate, acute cordate at buase, setose, pilose above, 2-6(-10) cm. across. Male flowers in fascicles. Pedicels 0.25-0.3 cm. long. Calyx 0.28-0.3 cm. long, hispid; lobes subulate. Corolla yellow, 0.5-0.6 cm. across; segmets ovate-rounded apiculate, hairy. Anthers with connective produced above the apex. Female flowers 1-2 together. Pedicels 0.2-0.5 cm. long. Ovary densely soft-hairy. Fruit ovoid-globose, green with white bands and hairy at first, turning to red on maturity, 1 to 2 seeded, 1 cm. long. Seeds 0.4-0.25 cm.

Plant occurring in the Upper Gangetic Plains, common. Herb common in roadsides, waste places, forest edges and grassy localities in Siwaliks range (Dehradun) and ascending the hills as far as subropical warmth extends. A common climber on shrubs and trees in northern region (Delhi) and adjacent areas.

Mukia scabrella Arns. with distribution in Asia, Africa and Australia; Herb. growing in Himachal Pradesh; Bhutan Plant found in orchards, Shimla. Flowering in June; ascending to 6,000 ft.

Zehneria umbellata Thwaites. with distribution in Asia, Africa, Australia and South america. Herb growing in Himachal PLradesh. Plant found commonly near Shimla and other areas.

Flowering in July - August. Plant ascending to 7,000 ft.

In Himachal Pradesh, the wild members of family Cucurbiaceae majorly include *Trichasnthes* and *Herpetospermum* and some other species (other than many usual cultivated genus and species). Particualrly the genera *Trichasanthes* and *Herpetoseprmum* are generally in valleys and other places, and they flower during the rainy season or around.

Important *Zehneria* species are following :

Zehneria scabra (Linn. f.) Sond.

Bryonia scabra L.f.

Zehneria hookeriana (W. & A.) Arn.

Melothria perpusilla (Bl.) Cogn.

Zeheria maysorensis var. **umbellata** (Chakr.) Kumari

Melothria mucrinata var. *umbellata* Chakr.

Zehneria thwaitesii (Schweinf.) Jaffrey.

Melothria thwaitesii (Jaffrey.

Melothria thwaitesii Schweinf.

M. zeylanica Cl.

Zehneria wallichii (Cl.) Jeffrey

Melothria wallichii Cl.

Zehneria indica (Lour.) Kern. - Arym.

Melothria indica Lour. excl syn. *M. regelii* Naudin

M. odorata Hook. f.

M. kucocarpa (Bl.) Cogn.

Zehneria maysorensis var. **umbellata** (Chakr.) Kumari

M. mucronata var. *umbellata* Chakr.

Zehneria maysorensis (W. & A.) Arn.

Z. baueriana sens Cl. non Edl. excl. syn. *Bryonia mucronata* Bl.

M. Melothria mucronata sensu Cogn. non *Bryonia mucrinata* Bl.

M. perpusilla (Bl.) Cogn. var. *subtruncata* Cogn.

Three relevant species of *Zeharia* Endl. in India particularly may be indicated :-

Zehneria baueriana Endl.

Z. mucronata Miq.

Bryonia mucronata Miq.

B. mysorensis Wall.

B. filliformis Roxb.

Karivia samoensis A. Crey.

Zehneria hookeriana Arn.

Zehneria umbellata Thwaites.

Similarly, the species of *Melothria* Linn. may be indicated:-

Melothria zeylanica C.B. Calrke

Bryonia deltoides Arn.

Aechmandra deltoides Arn.

Melothria wallichii C.B. Clarke.

Bryonia odorata Wall.

Melóthria indica Lour.

Bryonia tenella Roxb.

Aechmandra indica Arn.

M. rogelii Naud.

Melothria odorata Hk. f. & T.

Bryonia odorata Ham.

Genus *Solena* Loureiro in family Cucurbitaceae (about 110 genera and 640 species, chiefly in tropics, absent, in colder regions). with salient features - Slender climbers.

Tendrils simple. Leaves often lobed, cordate or sagitate. Inflorescence racemose, unbellate or flowers solitary. Calyx campanulate-tubular, 5-toothed. Corolla deeply partite. Stamens 3, free, inserted as the base of calyx, one 1-thecous two 2-thecous; anther cells weakly sigmoid, conactive produced or not, Pistillode trilbed. Staminodes 3. Ovary ovoid, with numerous horizontal ovules; style surrounded by a cupular disc at base; stigmas 3. Berry smooth; seeds turgid.

One or two species of *Solena* Lour. in tropical Asia and Malesia; perennial herbaceous climbers, found throughout India. Formerly included under *Zehneria* Endl. and or *Melothria* Linn. (sensu. lat.).

Genus *Mukia* Arnott in family Cucurbitaceae (about 37 genera and over 97 species in India) with salient features - Scandent or decumbent herbs. Tendrils simple. Leaves lobed, cordate. Flowers fascicled. Calyx campanulate, shortly 5-lobed. Corolla deeply partite. Stamens 3, free, inserted at the base of calyx, one 1-thecous, two 2-thecous; anther cells straight. Connective often produced. Pistillode small. Staminodes 3 or 0. Ovary ovid, hispid with numerous horizontal ovules; style surrounded by an annular disc at base; stigmas 2-3, papillose. Berry globose, smooth; seeds turgid, often scrobiculate, margined.

Four palaeotropical species; herbaceous climbers. Two species in India, one confined to Southern India and another occurs throughout India. Formerly included under *Melothria* Linn., an exclussively New World genus.

Genus *Zehneria* Enmdicher in family Cucurbitaceae (about 400 species in the warmer parts of world especially in the tropics) with salient features - Monoecious or dioecious climbers. Tendrils simple. Leaves cordate. Inflorescence an umbel, raceme, fascicle or of solitary flowers. Calyx campanulate, 5-toothed. Corolla 5-partite. Stamens 3 free, each 2 thecous, inserted at the throat of base of calyx tube; anthers cells arucate; connective not produced. Pistillode often 3-lobed. Staminodes 3. Ovary with few-many horizontal ovules; style surrounded by cupular disc; stigmas 3. Berry ovoid or globose; seeds often compressed.

Thirty palaeos tropical species; annual or perennial herbaceous climbers; five species in India, one ocurs throughout India, two in Southern India, with one extending to eastern Himalayas. Formerly treated under *Melothria* Linn.

Genus *Melothria* Linn. is distinguisable of style with an annular disc at the base; whereas the genus *Ctenolepis* Hook. f. style without a disc at the base and petiole with a stipule-like ciliate fruit; and these both genera have straight anther cells, but several other genera are with flexuose or conduplicate anther sells primarily, and other various characters of flowers, fruits, tendils and leaves mainly.

All the three relevant genera *Mukia* Arn., *Zehneria* Endl. and *Melothria* Linn. belong to group of genera having female flower mostly solitary, not in panicles and stamens 3 or 5, and specifically straight or arcuate anther cells, not 5 shaped; and individually the stamens 3 all 2-celled in *Zehnria* genus, when stamens 3, two 2-celled and one 1-celled in *Mukia* and *Solena* genera (also in some other genera), while anther cells are acruate in *Mukia*, and anther cells oblique and seeds turgid in *Solena* genus which differs from genus *Cucumis* Linn. having erect anther cells and compressed seeds.

These genera have entire petals, simple tendrils, calyx tubes not closed and bracts not spathaceous in general; and *Solena* has weakly sigmoid anthers and turgid seeds in particular. Specifically the stamens three, all 2-thecous and anthers acruate in *Zehneria;* and stamens 3, one 1-thecous in *Mukia;* and both genera have arcuate or straight anthers.

Solena heterophylla Lour. is very variable in shape, size, and degree of lobation of leaves, and size and shape of fruits found in the plants of species.

This species may closely resemble *Solena angulata* (Chakravarty) Babu syns. *Melothria angulata* Chakravarty., *Zehneria angulata* (Chakra.) Ellis. which appears to be variant of *Solena heterophylla* Lour. syn. *Zehneria umbellata* Thwaites, as its disgnostic characters like 9-angular fruits and strongly margined, rugose seeds are also found in the population of *Solena heterophylla* Lour. The characteristic features of *Solena angular* (Chakr.) Raizada show gradations which connects it with *Solena heterphylla* Lour, and also sometimes suggests it to be a form of *S. heterophylla* Lour.

Earlier, the three species of *Melothria* Linn. (generally now as distinct genera viz. *Melothria.*, *Zehneria* and *Solena*) carry difference primarily. For the instance, the male flowers in corymbs, connective of stamens not prolonged and seeds smooth are in *Melothria perpusilla* Cogn. and *Melothria heterophylla* Cogn. commonly, but the both species differ as former species has flowers monoecious, seeds small and much compressed, when flowers dioecious and seeds large turgid in latter species. Male flowers in clusters, connective of stamens produced and rough seeds in *Melothria maderaspatana* Cogn. which initially separates from previous species in characters of flowers, seeds and other features.

Zohenria maysorensis (Wight. & Arn.) Arn. is monoecious, and *Z. scabra* is dioecious. Three species *Zohneria mucronata, Z. scabra* and *Z. maysorensis,* latter two in India, may resemble *zehneria maysorensis* (W. & a.) Arn. Various species of *Zehneria* carry specific characterstics for distinction on the basis of flowers, fruits, leaves and tendrils, and other features.

Mukia maderaspatana (L.) Roemer is sometimes suggested to be monoecious taxa but its plants also have pistillate flowers or fruits and lack staminate flowers simaltaneously. *Mukia maderaspatana* syn. *M. scabrella* is also distinguishable from other genera like *Trichosenthes* Linn. and *Herpetospermum* Wall. ex Benth. in view of size of flowers firstly, as flowers more than 1 in. diam. in these (latter) genera, when the flowers of *Mukia* and *Zehneria* reduce to less than 1/4 in. diam.; and the two genera further differ. Stems and leaves rough, bristly or covered with minute sharp points in *Mukia* plants; whereas they are smooth, glabrous or slightly pubescent in Zehneria plants, alongwith other characterstics of distinction.

The roots, leasves, fruits and whole plant of *Solehna amplexicaulis* (Lamk.) Gandhi syn. *Melothria heterophylla* (Lour.) Cogn. are medicinally useful.

The juice of the roots are given with cumin and sugar in cold milk as a remedy for spermatorrhoea.

The juice of the leaves is applied parts which become inflamed from the application of the marking-nut juice. The root is considered stimulant, invigorating and purgative.

It is used for gonorrhoea and dysuria. The juice of the roots, mixed with cumin and sugar, is given in cold milk in cases of sepramatorrhoea, seminal weakness and other troubles. The juice is applied in the inflammation, erruptions and other complications caused with Bhallatakaphala svarasa, the fruit-secretion of *Smecarpus anacardium* Linn.

The seeds are used as a purgative.

The juice of leaves of the plant *Melothria indica.* Lour. is applied in sores of thrush and is used in the treatment of eye diasese.

Various parts of the plant *Solena* amplexicauils (Lamk.) Gandhi are used as medicine.

The fruits possess purgative properties.

The roots of the plant are useful as an antifertility drug and it is given to females in the form of powder or decoction for contraception.

The plant is considered a cooling. The leaves are made a paste and applied to cuts.

The leaves juice or powder is useful is antidiabetic remedy, and it is used in cases of diabetes, urinary troubles and particualrly diabetes inspidus.

The roots in powder form or as decoction is given in general debility and in other ailng conditions as a tonic.

The fruits are considered useful in fever as they carry antipyretic and diaphoretic activity.

The plant is considered useful in symphilis and stomach pains. It has stomachic activity and blood purifier.

The plant is useful in earache and labour pain. The juice is applied in form of drops in the condition of pain in ears and other allied complaints. Plant is considered helpful in labour stage for delivery.

The plant is exetrnally applied in the form of juice or pate in sores, wounds and ulces.

The plant is considered useful in paralytic disorders.

The seeds are useful against snake-bite.

The roots are considered useful as tonic drug, or as the restorative and fattening medicine. The roasted onions, gometta root, cummin, sugar and ghee are given, or gometta only with milk and sugar mixed ghee are given, or gometta only with milk and sugar are used for tonicity and restoration purpose.

The plant has utility as food or eatable item as the fruits are edible and relished. The ripe fruits are frequently utilised among the edible wild fruits. They also hold importance in the wild fruits of Cucurbitaceae which provides several cultigens for fruits and vegetables.

The ripe and unripe fruits both may be eaten, and frequently the ripen fruits are generally used. The roots asre also eaten after boiling or cooking.

The fruits are also eaten with that of *Capparis zeylanica* Linn. Fruits are also utilised as vegetable. The leaves are used as vegetable.

The brown colour fruits become red or bright red after they are matured, and these fruits are eaten with taste.

The fruits, roots and leaves are edible in different forms.

In veterinary medicine, the plant is medicinally useful. Plant is applied to sores of small pox in cattles.

The fruits, seeds, roots and whole plant of *Mukia maderaspatana* (L.) Cogn. syn. *Melothria scabrella* Arn. are medicinally useful.

The tender shoots and leaves are used as a gentle aperient, and recommended in vertigo and biliousness.

The seeds are crushed and applied on aching bodies, specially on strained backs.

The attractive berries are eaten by parots, the bulbul and other birds, and only the seeds that pass out of their stomach are said to germinate. The cattles like the plant but it is believed that the berries destroy the eyes, and hence its one of the local names (or some names indicate such meaning) which needs ascertainment.

The roots of the plant, when mascicasted, relieves the toothache. Decoction of roots is given in flatulence and similar abdominal troubles.

The plant is expectorant, the plant is used in compound preparation used for cough.

A decoction of seeds is useful as sudorfic medicine.

The decoction or powder of the seeds are useful in diarrhoea and diabetes.

The fruits are edible.

The fruits, leaves and plant of *Zehneria indica* (Lour) Kern. syn. *Melothria odorata* Hk. f. & Th., are medicinally useful.

The fruits are useful in stomach diseases.

The roots, fruits and plant of *Zehneria maysorensis* (Wt. & Arn.) Arn. syn. *Melothria nerpuailla* Cogn. are medicinally useful.

The roots are useful in veneral diseases.

Roots are used in preparation of sweet drink.

Fruits are edible and used as vegetable.

Whole plant of *Zehneria thwaitesii* (Scheein) Jeff. syn. *Melothria zeylanica* Cl. is medicinally useful.

The plant is edible.

The juice of the leaves of *Melothria indica* Lour. is applied in the sores of thrush. The juice is also used in treatment of eye disease.

The fruits of the plant possess purgative activity and used in constipation as a purgative medicine.

The roots of the plant *Melothria perpusilla* (Blume) Cogn. sysn. *Zehneria hookeriana* Arn. are used with milk in cases of fever and diarrhoea.

Medicinal properties and action of the plant dṛug - Rasa tikta-madhura, Vīrya uṣṇa, Vipāka kaṭu; Tridoṣasāmaka; and Karmas sāraka, mūtravirajanīya, sukrajanana, santatiniyamana, sītala, dāhasāmaka, maktastambhaka, balya, jvaraghna, sūlahar aktaprasādana - raktasodhaka, dīpana, sukhaprasavakara, vṛṣya, sothahara, ropana, wçakṣuṣya, mehahara, viṣaghna, rasāyana, medenāsaka, kaṭupauṣṭika, nāḍībalya,

Therapeutic indication for internal and external uses in jvasra, vibandha-koṣṭhabaddhatā, prameha-madhumeha, sukrameha, svapnadoṣa, viṣa, medoroga, daurbalya, viṣphota, sotha, dāha, tṛṣṇā, mūtraroga, kṣata, vraṇa, kaṇḍū, carmavikāra, ratijaroga, phiraṅga, kṣata, vraṇa, kaṇḍū, carmavikāra, ratijaroga, phiraṅga, karṇāsula, dantasula, āmāsayavikāRa, kaṣṭaprasava, sarpaviṣa-daṁsa, netraroga and pakṣāghāta.

Khādya - phala; (pakva) sāka - mūla, phala, patra.

Pasucikitsa - masurika pidika - vrana.

Gopāla karkaṭī, Vanakarkaṭa, the Sanskrit names for plant drug.

14

Xanthium strumarium Linn.

Xanthium indicum DC.

Family : Asterceae (Composiate)

Regional names : Chhota-gokhru (Hindi), Banokru (Bengal),Šhankeshwara (Bombay), Lanelsuru (Kashmiri), Sugglu (Punjabi), Maruluitge (Telgu), Marlumulla (Tamil); Chota-datura, Bhangra, Bichhu, Churchuta, Kutia, Kutta, Chirchita, Bhurat, Bhurchitta, Adasisi, Hurhurringa-ba, Kuthua, Latakni.

Erect, simple or branchd, aromatic, annual-biennial, robust herbs, up to 200 cm. tall. Stems furrowed, shortly pubescent, brown-blotched or-speckled. Leaves ovate-triangular, palmately 3 to 5-lobed or-angled, with a cuneate base, acute or acuminate, irregularly coarsely dentate, hispidulous, glandular, up to 10 X 12 cm. Petiole 2-30 cm. long. Heads solitary or fascicled, on short, laterial branches. Male heads short-peduncled, 0.3 cm. long, Involucral bracts 2 to 3-seriate, linear, acute, patent, ciliate, 0.25-0.3 cm., long. Pales spatulate, hairy at the top, 0.3 cm. long. Corolla greenish, 0.2-0.25 cm. long; lobes hairy. Female heads involucres finally 2-2.5 cm. (incl. 0.4-0.5 cm. long beaks) long, patent-hairy, with slightly incurved beaks and 0.3-0.5 cm. long prickles.

Distribution : Throughout the hotter parts of India and in the Himalayas up to 6,000 ft.

Flowering and fruiting : June to December

Xanthium strumarium Linn.

Unarmed coarse herb. Stem short, stout slightly branched, spotted, harsh with bristly hairs. Leaves petioled, 2-3 in. long, triangular-cordae, cuneate at the base; lobes toothed, undulate, scabrous on both sides. Heads in terminal and axillary racemes; barren, many, crowded at the top of the stem. Fruiting involucres 3/4 in. long, ovoid or oblong, covered with hooked prickles; beaks 2, erect.

Plant occurring common within the areas of Upper Gangetic Plains and adjacent sutropical Himalayas and Siwalik ranges Terai region. Plant often in waste places, along roadside ditches and near habitations, and various other places.

Xanthium strumarium Linn. Erect herbs up to 70 cm. Leaves broadly ovate, acute, 3-lobed, crenate, palmately veined, glandular. Involucre brown.

Tropics. Karnataka in India. Plant flowring in September.

Xanthium strumarium Linn. A scabrous erect herb or undershrub, up to 1 metre tall. Leaves triangular cordate, irregularly toothed. Heads bisexual and female (the latter 2-flowered) in racemes. Fruiting involucres clothed its hooked prickles.

Plant growing commonly in waste places, along roadsides and near populated areas, and occurring on the Ridge in disturbed areas; often gregarious; also found in low-lying areas, Delhi region and other adjacent areas, in northern India. Plant flowering and fruiting during the period from post-rains to summer seasons.

Genus *Xanthium* Linnaeus in the family Asteraceae (Asteraceae Dumort - Composiate Gische) with salient features - Annual herbs. Leaves alternate, petiolate, lobed, crenate, palmately veined. Heads monoecious discoid, with the functionally male heads in the upper axils, female heads in lower axils. Male head - bracts inseriate; receptacle, paleaceous; florets many, appeariing bisexual but achenes sterile, enclosed within pales style arms short, included. Feamle head globose, 2-florets, bracts all connate forming an indurate involucre which is riped by 2 spinescent hooks and covered by hooked spines; corolla; style arms exerted. Achenes 2, enclosed within the hardened spinescent involucre; pappus O.

There are 30 species of genus *Xanthium* Linn., distributed throughout the world; and 2 species naturalised throughout India, ascending upto 1,650 meters in the Himalayas. About 4 species probably all Americans; perhaps species indigenous to America, but now naturalised in India and various parts of Asia, and other warm regions.

Xanthium strumarium Linn. is most common species in the regions of occurrence, particualrly in waste places, road-sides, vacant lots or unused places and grounds, forest edges, forest clearings, scrub jungles, agricultural fields, tea plantations and near habitated areas in warm zones abundantly.

Plant is very variable in habit, hairiness, size and shape of leaves and inflorescence. It is distinct from *Xanthium inacquitatarum*. DC.

Genus *Xanthium* Linn. in the Tribe 5 Relianttheae of family Asteraceae (as in Tribe 3 Astereae but the style branches, each with a crown of hair below the stigma; receptacles with chaffy bracts) is specifically with the heads monoecious and achenes 2 to each head; when other genera are with heterogamous heads and achenes many to each head in the tribe genera having other various salient characters.

On the basis of flowers colour, the several genera may be grouped; and the genus *Xanthium* comes among the genera bearing white, whitish or creamy flowers, and particualrly simple heads, with male and female heads separate and the latter 2-flowered; as *Xanthium* falls in group of genera with corolla tubular, often ligualte in marginal flowers of radiate heads in non-lactiferous plants, and specifically homogamous heads, unisexual and female head 2-flowered, involucral bracts of female fl. connate into an elipsoid, firm, 2-locular body, covered with hooks, and bearing a bidentate beak on the apex of each cell; while various other genera have corolla ligulate in usually lactiferous plants with different in characters.

In two major group of genera having florets all tubular and (otherwise) ligulate, the plants glabrous, hairy or tomentose but not white-wholly, and leaves all alternate include genus *Xanthium* which is distincts of achenes enclosed in an indurate, spiny involucre, anthers and adherent in each other, and certain other characters.

The roots, fruits, leaves, seeds and whole plant of *Xanthium strumarium* Linn. are medicinally useful.

The roots are bitter, tonic and useful in strumous diseases and cancer. .

Plant is diaphoretic, sedative, sudorfic, sialogue, and considered useful in long-standing cases of malaria.

The fruits are cooling, demulcent and given in small-pox. Seeds of plant contains glycoside xanthostrumarin, oxalic acid; and also believed to have a second active principle.

Roots are useful for boils, cancer, wounds and ulcers.

Fruits are useful in eye diseases, and as colling medicine.

Leaves are useful in herpes, malaria, ringworm.

The fumes of seed sis useful in piles. Seeds oil is useful in rheumatism. Fruits are sudorfic. Leaves are useful in scrofula.

Plant is useful in urinary complaints.

The fruits and leaves are employed in drink.

Seedling is useful as a vegetable and cooking material.

The fruits are put in ear for hedache as a symbolic use.

Garland of fruits is made (after removing prickles) and used in night blindness as symbolic application.

Medicinal properties and action of the plant drug - Rasa Tikta-kaṣāya, Vīrya uṣṇa, Vipāka kaṭu, Tridoṣasāmaka; and Karma vraṇaropaṇa, arbudahara, jvaraghna, cakṣuṣya, tvacya, kaṇḍūghna, arsoghna, dadrughna, sothahara, vedanāsthapana, dantya, mutra-virajinīya, dāhasāmaka, balya, and sūlahara.

Therapeutic indication in Vraṇa, arbuda, karkaṭārbuda, viṣamajvasra, siraṅsūla, netraroga, arsa, āmavāta, dadru, dantasūla, mūtraroga, duṣṭavarṇa, dāha, carmavikāra and daurbalya, vātavyādhi, sandhisotha and various other ailments.

Khādya-peya-sāka - phala-patra-navapādapa (bāla)

Kaṇṭaphalā, the Sanskrit name for the plant drug.

Selected Bibliography

Duthie, J.F.: Flora of the Upper Gangetic Plain and of the Adjacement Siwalik and Sub-Himalayan tracts, Calcutta, 3 Vols, 1903-1929.

Hooker, J.D.: The Flora of British India, London, 7 Vols., 1872-1897.

Maheshwati, J.K.: The Flora of Delhi, New Delhi, 1963

Brandis, D.: The Forest Flora of North-West and Central, London, 1874

Dalzel, N.A. & Gibson, A.: The Bombay Flora, Bombay, 1861

Haines, H.H.: Supplement to Duthie's Flora of Upper Gangetic Plain, Dehradun, 1976

Cooke, T.: The Flora of the Presidency of Bombay, London, 2 vols., 1901-1908

Gamble, J.S. & Fisher, C.F.C. Flora of the Presidency of Madras, London, 11 parts, 1915-1936

Santapau, H.: The Flora of Saurastra, Rajkot, pt. 1, 1962

Stewart, J.L.: Punjab Plants, Lahore, 1869.

Saldanha, C.J. & Nicolson, D.H.: Flora of Hassan District, Karnataka, India, New Delhi, 1976

Chopra, R.N. et al: Glossary of Indian Medicinal Plants, New Delhi, 1956

Chiopra, R.N. et al: Supplement to Glossary of India Medicinal Plants, New Delhi, 1969

Kirtikar, K.R. & Basu, B.D.: Indian Medicinal Plants, 4 Vols., 1935

Bennet, S.S.R.: Name Changes in Flowering Plants of India and Adjacent Regions, Dehradun, 1987

Pandey, Gyanendra: Vanouṣadhi Manjūṣā-Maidānī Kṣetron Kī Upayogī Vanaspatiyān (by Prof. Ram Nath Vaidya), Hardwar, 1990

Witt, D.O.: Forest Flora of Berar Circle, Nagpur, 1958

Waheedkhan, M.A.: Madhya Pradesh Plants, Forest Deptt., M.P. Rewa, 1971

Watt, G.: A Dictionary of the Economic Products of India, Vols., Dehradun, 1889-1972

Anonymous: Wealth of India (Raw Materials), 10 Vols. (8), New Delhi, 1948-1956-1969

Anonymous: Medicinal Plants of India, Vol. I, I.C.M.R., New Delhi, 1976

Babu, C.R.: Herbaceous Flora of Dehradun, New Delhi, 1977

Pandey, Gyanendra: Medicinal Flowers: Puṣpāyurveda Medicinal Flowers of India and Adjacent Regions, Delhi, 1992

Brandis, D.: Indian Trees, London, 1906

Hara, H. et al: The Flora of Eastern Himalayas, Tokyo, 1966

Kanjilal, U.N. et la: Flora of Assam, 7 Vols., Shilong, 1934-1940

Nadkarni, K.M.: Indian Materia Medica, Vol. 2, Bombay, 1954

Pandey, Gyanendra: Gyanendra Enumeratio Plantamedica, (Ed. - Sumitra Pandey) Delhi, 1993

Prain, D.: Bengal Plants, Vols. 1-2, Calcutta, 1963

Bamber, C.J.: Plants of the Punjab, Lahore, 1916

Boddome, R.H.: The Flora Sylvatica for Southern India, Madras, 2 Vols., 1860-1874

Hutchinson, J. & Dalzel, J.M.: Flora of West Tropical Flora, London, 1954-1958

Kitamura, S.: Flora of Afghanistan, Japan, 1960

Kurz, S.: Forest Flora of British Burma, Calcutta, 2 Vols., 1877

Parker, R.N.: A Forest Flora for the Punjab with Hazara and Delhi, Lahore, 1918

Santapau, H.: The Flora of Khandala on the Western Ghats of India, RBST, 1953 (ed. 1960)

Merrill, E.D.: An Enumeration of Philippine Flowering Plants, 4 Vols., Manila, 1923-1926

Oliver, D. et al: Flora of Tropical Africa, Vols. 1-10, Part 1, London, 1868-1937

Samtapau, H.: Flora of Saurastra, Part I, Rajkot, 1962

Van, Steens, C.G.G.J.: Flora of Malesiana, Vols. 4-5, 1948-1958

Jain, S.K.: Dictionary of Indian Folk Medicine and Ethnobotany, New Delhi, 1991

Sharma, P.V.: Dravyaguna Vigyan, Varanasi, 1956

Vaidya, B.G.: Nighantu Adarsha, Vol.I, Varanasi, 1968

Singh, B. et al: Glossary of Vegetable Drugs in Brhattrayi, Varanasi, 1962

Kanjilal, U.: Forest Flora of Chakrata, Dehradun and Saharanpur Dorest divisions, Dehradun, 1969

Chopra, R.N. et.al: Poisonous Plants of India, Delhi, 1949

Lewis, F.: The Vegetable Products of Ceylon, Colombo, 1934

Burkill, I.H.: A Dictionary of the Economic Products of the Malay Peninsula, London, Vols. 2, 1935

Singh, H.B. et al: Wild Edible Plants of India, IBPGR, ICAR, New Delhi, 1978

Ambasta, S.P.: Useful Plants of India, CSTE, New Delhi, 1986

Perry, L.M.: Medicinal Plants of East and Southeast Asia, Massachusetts, 1980

Bhandari, M.M.: Flora of Indian Desert, Jodhpur, 1978

Chowdhery, H.J. et al: Flora of Himachal Pradesh, BSI, Calcutta, 3 Vols., 1984

Haridas, K.et al: Forest Flora of Meghalaya, Vols. 1-2, Dehradun, 1985

Shah, G.L.: Flora of Gujarat State, Vols. 2, Ballabha Vidyanagar, 1978

Henry, A.N. et al: Flora of Tamilnadu, 3 Vols., B.S.I., Calcutta, 1989

Singh, A.N. et al: Dictionary of Economic Plaints of India, I.C.A.R., New Delhi, 11965

Bennet, S.S.R.: Flora of Howrah District, Calcutta, 1979

Duke, J.A.: Isthmian Ethnobotanical Dictionary, Jodhpur, 1986, 3rd. Ed.

Oommachan, M.: Flora of Bhopal, Bhopal, 1977

Deb, D.B.: The Flora of Tripura State, 2 Vols., New Delhi, 1981

Singh, D.J.: Unani Dravyaguna Vigyan, Vol. Part III, Lucknow, 1978

Acharya, Y.T.: Dravyaguna Vigyanam, Vol. II, Part II, Bombay, 1950

Singh, R.S.: Vanaoudhadhi Nidarshika-Ayurvedic Pharmacopoeia, Lucknow, 1969

Dwivedi, V.N.: Ausadhi Vigyan Sahstra-Ayurvedic Pharmacology, Nagpur, 1970

Stafleu, F.A.: Taxonomic Literature, Utrecht-Netherlands & Zug-Switzerland, 1967

Osamsten, A.E.: Forest Flora of Kumaon, Allahabad, 1927

Collett, H.: Flora of Simalensis, Calcutta, 1921

Nath, B. et al: Important Ayurvedic Plants of Madhya Pradesh, M.P. Govt., Rewa, 1968

Santapau, H. et al: A Dictionary of the Flowering Plants in India, C.S.I.R., New Delhi, 1973

Haridasan, K. et al: Forest of Meghalaya, Vols. 2, Dehradun, 1985

Dey, A.C.: Indian Medicinal Plants, Dehradun, 1980

Husain, A. et al: Dictionary of Indian Medicinal Plants, CIMAP, Lucknow, 1992

Thakur, R.S. et al: Major Medicinal Plants of India, CIMAP, Lucknow, 1992

Rao, R.S.: Flora of Goa, Diu, Daman, Dada and Nagarhaveli, B.S.I., 2 Vols., Calcutta, 1985-86

Shelly, B.V. et al: Flora of Rajasthan, Vol.I. B.S.I., Calcutta, 1987

Sharma, B.M. et al: Flora of Jammu and Plants of Neighbourhood, Vol., Dehradun, 1981

Kihara, H.: Fauna and Flora of Nepal Himalayas, Kyoto, Japan, 1955

Hutchinson, J.: The Genera of Flowering Plants, Oxford, 1964

---

* Incorporating classical treatises and other works (medicine, materia medica and allied branches) in texts; and the periodicals.

Indices

1. Index to Botanical names
2. Index to Sanskrit Names
3. Index to Regional Names

Index-1

Botanical Names

B. penangiana Hook. f.
B. scandens Roxb.
B. scandens Willd.
B. montana Willd.
B. montana var. communis Prain.
B. montana Royle.
B. squamosa (Lamk.) Gaertn.
B. stipularis Blume.
B. crenulata Blume.
B. ovata var. crustisii (Hook. f.) Airy-Shaw.
B. retusa var. roxburghiana Muell.
B. spinosa Willd.
B. assamica Hook. f.

Cissus araneosus Dalz. & Gibs.
Clerodendron spicatum Thunb.
C. serratum (L.) Moon.
Clerodendrum multiflorum (Burm. f.) Kuntze.
C. phlomidis Linn. f.
C. viscosum Vent.
C. infortunatum auct. non. L.
C. infortunatum Linn.
C. castaneaefoium Klotzech.
Cardus radicans Roxb.
C. rambus Roxb.
Centaurea divaricata Vahl.
Caesalpinia digyama Rottl.
Cnicus angustifolius Wall.
Cicendra hyssopifolia W. & A.
Caesalpinia oleosperma Roxb.
Corralocarpus epigeus C.B. Clarke
Convovulus candicans Wall.
C. hypocuatiformis Desv.
Croton hastatus L.
Claxylon mercurialis Thw.
Cochleospermum religiosum Altton.

C. gossypium DC.
Craterostigma plantaginea (Benth.) Hoochchst.

Dicoma lanuginosa DC.
D. tonetosa Cass.
Doronicum calcaratub Roxb.

Glossostylis arvensis Benth.
Gentiana verticillata L.

Hippion orientale Dalz.
Hymenospermus dentuonum Benth.

Inula indica L.
I. indica Willd.
I. vestita Wall.

Lamprachaenum microcephalum Benth.
Lettsomia uniflora Roxb.
L. ornata Roxb.

Micrococa morcurialis (Linn.) Benth.
Microlonchus divaricatus DC.
Melasma avense (Benth.) Hand.-Maza.
M. indicum (Benth.) Wettst. var. monticolum Engl.

Ocimum tuberosum Roxb.
O. aristatum Bl.
O. thymiflorus (Benth.) Sleeren.
Oligochaeta ramosa (Roxb.) Wagenitz.
Onopordon lanatum Herb.
Orthosiphon pallidus Royle ex Benth.
O. stamineus Benth.
O. viscosus Benth.
O. glabratus Benth.
O. grandiflorus Boddings.

O. rubicundus (D. Don.) Bentham.
Oentanema radiatum Boiss.

P. vestita (Wall.) DC.
Plectranthes rubicundus D.Don.
Pentanema indicus (L.) Ling.

Rivea fragrans Nimmo.
R. hypocrateriformis (Desr.) Choisy.
R. ornata Aitch.
R. laoticaossuisetn.
R. ornata var. griffthii Clarke.

Sauromattum venosum (Ait.) Kunth.
S. pedatum (Willd.) Schott.
S. guttatum (Wall.) Schott.
Stctophyllum glabrum Edgew.
Slevotia verticillata Benth.

Tragia involucrata Linn.
T. cannabina Linn.
T. hispida Willd.
T. mercurialis (Liin.) Benth.
T. muellirima var. cordata (Muell-Arg) Pax & Hoffman
T. pleukonetii A.R. Smith
T. canabina Linn. f.
T. involucrata var. angustifolia Hook. f.
T. involucurta var. canabina Muell-Arg.
T. muelleriana var. cordata Muell-Arg.
Tridax procumbens Linn.
Tricholepis grlaberima DC.
T. stictophyllum Clarke.
T. radicans (Roxb.) DC.
Typhonium trilobatum Schott.
T. scamense Engler.
T. orixens Schott.
T. triste Griff.
Tubiflora acaulis O. Kuntze.

Vitex negundo Linn.
Vicoa indica (W.) DC.
V. cassii
V. auriculata Cass
Ventilago denticulata Willd.
V. calyculata Tulsene
V. madraspatana Gaertn. var. calyculata (Tab.) King.
V. bracteata Wall.
V. micrantha Tulasne.
Volutarella divaricata (DC.) Benth.
V. ramosa (Roxb.) Sant.
Volkameria infortunata Roxb.
Vitis erioclada W. & A.
V. indica W. & A.
V. rugosa Wall.
V. tomentosa Heyne ex Rlth.
V. indica sensu Waidon.
V. araneosus (Dalz. & Gibs.) Lawson.
V. cinnamomia Wall.
V. latifolia Roxb.
V. montana Lawson.

Yeropappus lanugginosus Wall.

Index 2

Sanskrit Names

Mulanatrā
Mārakava

Nīlimā
Nīlapuṣpī
Nāhīkanda
Nirguṇḍī
Nirguṇḍī Vandaka-bandāka
Nirguṇḍībhava bandāka

Pattanga
Phaṅjī
Pītabhṇgarāja
Paṣāṇasāka
Pādaprasarī

Raktarodhī
Rakta-vajra-kanda

Sukanasā
Suphalinī
Surendrakanda
Sahasramūlā
Svetakuṭheraka

Tāmravallī

Vaṭa oatra
Vandhyāvarī
Vajrakanda
Vajraproktā
Vātanirmūlikā
Vṛṣcikālī
Vāmatarunī (Rāmataruṇī)

Index-3

Regional Names

Gadhvi
Gurrpukattiyaku
Gundar
Genjra
Geng
Gengal
Ganjlay
Ganeri
Gudpasari
Gurhmi
Ghamra
Gada
Ghatkacchu

Hasualarang
Homuli
Haranacana

Jangali-amgur
Kamraja
Karantavalli
Kattukkadimundirigi
Kumarlai
Khaja
Kaj
Kaja
Kantakoi
Karganalia
Kaishe
Kaur
Kadu
Kalibasut
Kendagogu
Katira
Kadhayo
Kumbhi
Kumbi

Khirkand
Kuktupita
Kalibel
Kuriyadai
Kanyel
Kevli
KandageddaKarunaikhihangue
Kammichi
Kidura
Kadvinayi
Kadvinahi
Kararinai
Kollemhavekiichauna

Loth
Lakhandi

Midaki
Musal
Motabor
Muchuttal
Mirchiakand
Mullavenagi
Mukhayini

Nathagidu
Nilphuli
Nilam
Nirganga
Nunegacha
Niladambu
Nahi
Nilakadambu
Nagandha bavari
Navananabjichapla

Osari

Puchidita
Pumpilu
Panibel
Phatarpod
Pantegi
Perugilai
Peruku
Pumiaye
Pilikapas
Patharsaga
Patharchata
Palanidardu
Parh
Phang
Phand
Phanji
Pirahdandi
Pinchuli
Pitti
Pappili
Pappali

Randraksha
Raidhuti
Raidhani
raktapita

Sirunaralai
Sing
Sakagi
Sasamula
Sambarvalli
Semparavalli

Tambacco
Tamakhu
Turachi
Tanukupututti

Uchunti
Umulguchi
Utateri Fusiyani

Vakerimula
Vekri mula
Vengaimaram
Vakribhayu
Vakeri
Vakeri ca bhata
Vallari
Vamanadandi

General Index to Medicinal Plants*

* List denoting number(s) of section : plant(s) group.